CONTENTS

ONE YEAR LATER: EVALUATING THE EFFECTIVENESS OF PROJECT BIOSHIELD

HEARING

BEFORE THE

COMMITTEE ON GOVERNMENT REFORM

HOUSE OF REPRESENTATIVES

ONE HUNDRED NINTH CONGRESS

FIRST SESSION

JULY 14, 2005

Serial No. 109–59

Printed for the use of the Committee on Government Reform

Available via the World Wide Web: http://www.gpoaccess.gov/congress/index.html
http://www.house.gov/reform

U.S. GOVERNMENT PRINTING OFFICE

23–143 PDF WASHINGTON : 2005

For sale by the Superintendent of Documents, U.S. Government Printing Office
Internet: bookstore.gpo.gov Phone: toll free (866) 512–1800; DC area (202) 512–1800
Fax: (202) 512–2250 Mail: Stop SSOP, Washington, DC 20402–0001

COMMITTEE ON GOVERNMENT REFORM

TOM DAVIS, Virginia, *Chairman*

CHRISTOPHER SHAYS, Connecticut
DAN BURTON, Indiana
ILEANA ROS-LEHTINEN, Florida
JOHN M. McHUGH, New York
JOHN L. MICA, Florida
GIL GUTKNECHT, Minnesota
MARK E. SOUDER, Indiana
STEVEN C. LATOURETTE, Ohio
TODD RUSSELL PLATTS, Pennsylvania
CHRIS CANNON, Utah
JOHN J. DUNCAN, JR., Tennessee
CANDICE S. MILLER, Michigan
MICHAEL R. TURNER, Ohio
DARRELL E. ISSA, California
GINNY BROWN-WAITE, Florida
JON C. PORTER, Nevada
KENNY MARCHANT, Texas
LYNN A. WESTMORELAND, Georgia
PATRICK T. McHENRY, North Carolina
CHARLES W. DENT, Pennsylvania
VIRGINIA FOXX, North Carolina
——— ———

HENRY A. WAXMAN, California
TOM LANTOS, California
MAJOR R. OWENS, New York
EDOLPHUS TOWNS, New York
PAUL E. KANJORSKI, Pennsylvania
CAROLYN B. MALONEY, New York
ELIJAH E. CUMMINGS, Maryland
DENNIS J. KUCINICH, Ohio
DANNY K. DAVIS, Illinois
WM. LACY CLAY, Missouri
DIANE E. WATSON, California
STEPHEN F. LYNCH, Massachusetts
CHRIS VAN HOLLEN, Maryland
LINDA T. SANCHEZ, California
C.A. DUTCH RUPPERSBERGER, Maryland
BRIAN HIGGINS, New York
ELEANOR HOLMES NORTON, District of Columbia
———
BERNARD SANDERS, Vermont (Independent)

MELISSA WOJCIAK, *Staff Director*
DAVID MARIN, *Deputy Staff Director/Communications Director*
ROB BORDEN, *Parliamentarian*
TERESA AUSTIN, *Chief Clerk*
PHIL BARNETT, *Minority Chief of Staff/Chief Counsel*

ONE YEAR LATER: EVALUATING THE EFFECTIVENESS OF PROJECT BIOSHIELD

THURSDAY, JULY 14, 2005

HOUSE OF REPRESENTATIVES,
COMMITTEE ON GOVERNMENT REFORM,
Washington, DC.

The committee met, pursuant to notice, at 11:30 a.m., in room 2154, Rayburn House Office Building, Hon. Tom Davis (chairman of the committee) presiding.

Present: Representatives Davis of Virginia, Shays, Waxman, Issa, Foxx, Maloney, Cummings, Kucinich, Davis of Illinois, Clay, Watson, Van Hollen, Ruppersberger, and Norton.

Staff present: Melissa Wojciak, staff director; David Marin, deputy staff director/communications director; Keith Ausbrook, chief counsel; Rob White, press secretary; Drew Crockett, deputy director of communications; Edward Kidd and Susie Schulte, professional staff members; John Brosnan, GAO detailee; Teresa Austin, chief clerk; Sarah D'Orsie, deputy clerk; Kristina Sherry, legislative assistant; Leneal Scott, computer systems manager; Josh Sharfstein, minority health policy advisor; Robin Appleberry, minority counsel; Earley Green, minority chief clerk; and Jean Gosa, minority assistant clerk.

Chairman TOM DAVIS. The committee will come to order. I want to welcome everybody to today's oversight hearing to assess the implementation of Project BioShield thus far. The purpose of this hearing is to consider whether the Project BioShield program is being adequately implemented to accelerate the research, development and purchase of effective countermeasures against agents of bioterrorism.

Now that the Department of Health and Human Services has begun to utilize its special authorities granted by Congress through the Project BioShield Act of 2004, the committee feels it is time to review how these authorities are being executed. Specifically, the committee will consider whether adequate medical countermeasures to protect our population against a biological attack are being procured.

As we tragically learned during the fall of 2001, our Nation is vulnerable to biological terrorism. Letters laced with anthrax caused the deaths of five individuals. Thousands more had to be treated. The death toll could have been higher if there had not been effective countermeasures to treat that particular form of anthrax.

The Project BioShield Act of 2004 gave the Federal Government better tools to develop and purchase vaccines and other drugs to protect Americans in the event of bioterrorist attacks. If the United States were to be attacked with these deadly pathogens, the need for the corresponding vaccines, tests and treatments would be widespread and immediate.

The Government has made some progress over the past year in implementing the BioShield program and improving preparedness efforts against bioterrorism. To date, DHS and HHS have determined that anthrax, botulinum toxins, smallpox and radiological and nuclear agents pose a significant material threat to Americans and to U.S. national security. Health and Human Services has solicited and awarded contracts for medical countermeasures against these threats.

In November 2004, HHS awarded a contract to VaxGen for up to 75 million doses of a new generation anthrax rPA vaccine, and in May awarded a contract for 5 million doses of the existing FDA-licensed anthrax vaccine produced by BioPort Corp. Additionally, HHS awarded a contract for pediatric potassium iodide in March of this year for inclusion within the Strategic National Stockpile.

But in spite of these efforts, there remains some concern as to HHS's moving too slowly to award contracts. Among the questions we are going to ask today: How do we prepare against the threat of bioterrorism while waiting for new countermeasures to be researched and developed? Are we adequately linking threat assessments to the procurement of appropriate countermeasures? And most importantly, are we safer now than we were before BioShield was enacted?

Witnesses on our second panel are going to express their concerns over the transparency of the solicitation process and whether companies are fully aware of how they are being evaluated and what certain terms and criteria are considered when HHS responds to a solicitation. We will also hear concerns about whether the implementation of BioShield is working to erase barriers to entry to the bio-defense market and if more incentives are needed.

I look forward to a robust discussion on whether the procurement of medical countermeasures to date has been sufficient and how best do we work toward improvements necessary for even greater preparedness.

Project BioShield needs to work. It was crafted so that the United States could better harness the power of the commercial marketplace to protect our citizens against threats, whether they be nuclear, biological or radiological, or whatever.

Just 1 week after terrorists detonated four bombs in the heart of London, taking the lives of more than 50 people, no one should need a reminder of how real these threats are. Anyone who has read the 9/11 Commission report or who has been listening to the experts who have studied these issues in depth can't help but understand this.

I want to show a short video that is illustrative.

[Video shown.]

Chairman TOM DAVIS. The only drug we have right now is potassium iodide in case of a nuclear attack. But we need the development of better, next generation treatment of drugs and where are we?

This is not an academic exercise. Project BioShield was conceived to help us face the most pressing threats facing our Nation today, and we need it to live up to that promise. There was a consensus in the Presidential race that this is an area we need to proceed in. And yet to date we have not seen the kind of progress, I think, that the act wanted and that Congress demands and the American people need.

We have a great selection of witnesses today and I look forward to their testimony. But before that, I would like to recognize our distinguished ranking member, Mr. Waxman, for his opening statement.

[The prepared statement of Chairman Tom Davis follows:]

Opening Statement of Chairman Tom Davis
Committee on Government Reform
"One Year Later: Evaluating the Effectiveness of Project BioShield"
July 14, 2005

Good morning. I want to welcome everyone to today's oversight hearing to assess the implementation of Project BioShield thus far. The purpose of this hearing is to consider whether the Project BioShield program is being adequately implemented to accelerate the research, development, and purchase of effective countermeasures against agents of bioterrorism.

Now that the Department of Health and Human Services (HHS) has begun to utilize its special authorities granted by Congress through the Project BioShield Act of 2004, the Committee feels it is time to review how these authorities are being executed. Specifically, the Committee will consider whether adequate medical countermeasures to protect our population against a biological attack are being procured.

As we tragically learned during the fall of 2001, our nation is vulnerable to biological terrorism. Letters laced with anthrax caused the deaths of five individuals, and thousands more had to be treated. The death toll could have been higher if there had not been effective countermeasures to treat that particular form of anthrax.

The "Project BioShield Act of 2004" gave the federal government better tools to develop and purchase vaccines and other drugs to protect Americans in the event of a bioterrorist attack. If the United States were to be attacked with these deadly pathogens, the need for the corresponding vaccines, tests, and treatments would be widespread and immediate.

The government has made some progress over the past year in implementing the BioShield program and improving preparedness efforts against bioterrorism. To date, DHS and HHS have determined that anthrax, botulinum toxins, smallpox, and radiological and nuclear agents pose a significant material threat to Americans and to U.S. national security. HHS has solicited and awarded contracts for medical countermeasures against these threats. In November 2004, HHS awarded a contract to VaxGen for up to 75 million doses of a new generation anthrax rPA vaccine, and in May awarded a contract for 5 million doses of the existing FDA licensed anthrax vaccine produced by BioPort Corporation. Additionally, HHS awarded a contract for pediatric potassium iodine in March of this year for inclusion within the Strategic National Stockpile.

In spite of these efforts, there remains some concern that HHS is moving too slowly to award contracts and has made insufficient efforts to stockpile existing countermeasures while new and improved ones are being developed. Among the questions we will ask today: How do we prepare against the threat of bioterrorism while waiting for new countermeasures to be researched and developed? Are we adequately linking threat assessments to the procurement of appropriate countermeasures? And, most importantly, are we safer now that we were before BioShield was enacted?

Witnesses on our second panel may raise concerns over the transparency of the solicitation process and whether companies are fully aware of how they are being evaluated and what certain terms and criteria are considered when HHS responds to a solicitation. We will also hear concerns today about whether the implementation of BioShield is working to erase barriers of entry to the bio-defense market and if more incentives are needed. I look forward to a robust discussion on whether the procurement of medical countermeasures to date has been sufficient and how best to work towards the improvements necessary for even greater preparedness.

Project BioShield needs to work. It was crafted so that the United States could better harness the power of the commercial marketplace to protect its citizens against threats, whether they be nuclear, or biological, or radiological, or what have you.

And, just one week after terrorists detonated four bombs in the heart of London, taking the lives of more than 50 people, no one should need a reminder of how real these threats are. Anyone who has read the 9/11 Commission Report, or has been listening to the experts who have studied these issues in depth, cannot help but understand this. I'd like to show a short video that is illustrative.

[SHOW VIDEO]

This is not an academic exercise. Project BioShield was conceived to help us face the most pressing threats facing our nation today, and we need it to live up to that promise. We have a fine selection of witnesses today and I look forward to their testimony.

Mr. WAXMAN. Thank you very much, Mr. Chairman.

I think we owe it to our audience to explain that we were late in coming to the hearing today partly due to the chairman's efforts because there was a vote on the House floor where almost all of the Members had voted aye, the chairman was among a few that voted no. When people looked and saw his "no" vote, little by little they changed their aye to no, and the matter that was on the floor ready to pass was defeated. So the chairman is clearly a very strong leader, both on the House floor and in this committee.

Chairman TOM DAVIS. You can have as much time as you want today, Mr. Waxman. [Laughter.]

Mr. WAXMAN. One year ago, Congress passed legislation to establish Project BioShield. This important program seeks to encourage private companies to develop innovative drugs, vaccines and other measures to address bioterrorist threats. The plan is for these products to be delivered to the American people in an emergency by a fully functional public health system. Today's hearing is an opportunity to assess how Project BioShield is working. It is also an opportunity to ask whether the rest of our public health system is prepared to do its part of the job.

The answer is not encouraging. While Congress has provided guaranteed funding for BioShield, the administration has repeatedly shortchanged core public health services. This failure threatens our ability to respond to serious biological threats, whether natural or man-made.

Two weeks ago, our committee learned that the United States is unprepared for a flu pandemic which could claim as many as 500,000 American lives. Unlike other nations, our plan to respond to a flu pandemic is not finalized. We have not purchased the antiviral medication we need. We do not have adequate supplies of vaccine. And yet the administration has refused to admit the obvious: extra funding is needed to do the right job.

There are also large gaps in our state of preparedness for a bioterrorist attack. Only a handful of States have the capacity to deliver essential medications and vaccines contained in the Strategic National Stockpile to their citizens. There is no point in having a new anthrax vaccine or nerve gas antidote if the people whose lives are at risk cannot obtain treatment in time.

But rather than shore up the system to deliver these products, the administration has proposed cutting $130 million from State and local health departments. While BioShield offers promise for the future, the administration's chronic under-funding of public health is risking our ability to respond to a crisis in the meantime. The only maker of the current smallpox vaccine in the United States may close its production facility because the administration is failing to invest in ongoing production capacity. Similarly, the only maker of a licensed anthrax vaccine has said it may be forced to close its doors without a Government contract to keep its machines running.

Until new and improved products are actually available, it makes no sense to lose access to current products that are protecting the American people.

The weaknesses in the public health system are even undermining the ability of Project BioShield to succeed in developing new, cutting edge products. In announcing the President's proposal, the White House stated that Project BioShield would "ensure resources to develop next generation countermeasures." The proposal was billed as a measure to speed research and develop medical countermeasures based on the most promising recent scientific discoveries. But the latest BioShield contract uses more than $120 million for the procurement of an anthrax vaccine that was licensed in 1970, 35 years ago.

Now, let me be clear. I am not against, in fact I do support the purchase of existing anthrax vaccine. But such a purchase should be made with public health funds, not with the special pool of resources set aside by Congress to encourage research into groundbreaking new products.

BioShield was supposed to be a shot in the arm for public health readiness, but it is being used as a crutch. Today we will discuss some of the nuts and bolts of BioShield. There are important questions about how the program is working to encourage new products, balancing the needs of business with responsibility to the taxpayer.

We shouldn't lose sight of what BioShield is all about: a safer America. We need not only a better BioShield but also a system that can support and deliver the best possible response to public health emergencies. We must demand that the administration and Congress put all the resources that are necessary into this effort.

I am pleased that some of our Nation's leaders in public health preparedness are here today. I want to thank them for their efforts on behalf of the American people. I look forward to all of the testimony from today's witnesses.

[The prepared statement of Hon. Henry A. Waxman follows:]

Statement of
Rep. Henry A. Waxman, Ranking Minority Member
Committee on Government Reform
Hearing on
One Year Later: Evaluating the Effectiveness of Project BioShield

July 14, 2005

One year ago, Congress passed legislation to establish Project Bioshield. This important program seeks to encourage private companies to develop innovative drugs, vaccines, and other measures to address bioterrorist threats. The plan is for these products to be delivered to the American people in an emergency by a fully functional public health system.

Today's hearing is an opportunity to assess how Project Bioshield is working. It is also an opportunity to ask whether the rest of our public health system is prepared to do its part of the job.

The answer is not encouraging.

While Congress has provided guaranteed funding for Bioshield, the Administration has repeatedly shortchanged core public health services. This failure threatens our ability to respond to serious biological threats, whether natural or man-made.

Two weeks ago, our Committee learned that the United States is unprepared for a flu pandemic, which could claim as many as 500,000 American lives. Unlike other nations, our plan to respond to a flu pandemic is not finalized. We have not purchased the antiviral medication we need. We do not have adequate supplies of vaccine. And yet the Administration has refused to admit the obvious: Extra funding is needed to do the job right.

There are also large gaps in our state of preparedness for a bioterrorist attack. Only a handful of states have the capacity to deliver essential medications and vaccines contained in the strategic national stockpile to their citizens. There is no point in having a new anthrax vaccine or nerve gas antidote if the people whose lives are at risk cannot obtain treatment in time. But rather than shore up the system to deliver these products, the Administration has proposed cutting $130 million from state and local health departments.

While Bioshield offers promise for the future, the Administration's chronic underfunding of public health is risking our ability to respond to a crisis in the meantime. The only maker of the current smallpox vaccine in the United States may close its production facility because the Administration is failing to invest in ongoing production capacity.

Similarly, the only maker of licensed anthrax vaccine has said that it may be forced to close its doors without a government contract to keep its machines running. Until new and improved products are actually available, it makes no sense to lose access to current products that are protecting the American people.

The weaknesses in the public health system are even undermining the ability of Project Bioshield to succeed in developing new, cutting-edge products. In announcing the President's proposal, the White House stated that Project BioShield would "ensure resources to develop next-generation countermeasures." The proposal was billed as a measure to "speed research and development on medical countermeasures based on the most promising recent scientific discoveries." But the latest Bioshield contract uses more than $120 million for the procurement of an anthrax vaccine that was licensed in 1970 – 35 years ago.

Let me be clear that I support the purchase of the existing anthrax vaccine. But such a purchase should be made with public health funds, not with the special pool of resources set aside by Congress to encourage research into groundbreaking new products.

Bioshield was supposed to be a shot in the arm for public health readiness, but it is being used as a crutch.

Today, we will discuss some of the nuts and bolts of Bioshield. There are important questions about how the program is working to encourage new products, balancing the needs of businesses with responsibility to the taxpayer.

But we must not lose sight of what Bioshield is all about – a safer America. We need not only a better Bioshield, but also a system that can support and deliver the best possible response to public health emergencies. We must demand that the Administration and Congress put all the resources that are necessary into this effort.

I am pleased that some of our nation's leaders in public health preparedness are here today. I thank you for your efforts on behalf of the American people. I look forward to all of the testimony from today's witnesses.

Chairman TOM DAVIS. Thank you.

I want to again thank everybody for your patience in being with us today. We had some votes right after 10 a.m., and as Mr. Waxman alluded, one vote took a little longer than normal. I am not sure that it was my stellar "no" vote up there that switched everybody else, but about 100 Members came in, I think they read the amendment after they voted and decided to switch.

Members will have 7 days to submit written statements. Is there anyone else who wants to make an opening statement? Without objection, they will all be in the record.

We have today the Honorable Stewart Simonson, the Assistant Secretary for Public Health Emergency Preparedness, Department of Health and Human Services; Dr. Anthony Fauci, the Director of the National Institute of Allergy and Infectious Diseases, National Institutes of Health; and Dr. John Vitko, the Director of Biological Countermeasure Portfolio, Science and Technology Directorate, Department of Homeland Security.

It is our policy, as you know, we swear you in before you testify. So if you would just rise and raise your right hands.

[Witnesses sworn.]

Chairman TOM DAVIS. Mr. Simonson, we will start with you and we will move straight down. Your entire statement is a part of the record, and our questions are based on your entire written testimony. Thanks for your patience.

STATEMENTS OF STEWART SIMONSON, ASSISTANT SECRETARY, OFFICE OF PUBLIC HEALTH EMERGENCY PREPAREDNESS, U.S. DEPARTMENT OF HEALTH AND HUMAN SERVICES; ANTHONY S. FAUCI, M.D., DIRECTOR, NATIONAL INSTITUTE OF ALLERGY AND INFECTIOUS DISEASES, NATIONAL INSTITUTES OF HEALTH; AND JOHN VITKO, JR., M.D., DIRECTOR, BIOLOGICAL COUNTERMEASURES PORTFOLIO, SCIENCE AND TECHNOLOGY DIRECTORATE, DEPARTMENT OF HOMELAND SECURITY

STATEMENT OF STEWART SIMONSON

Mr. SIMONSON. Good morning, Chairman Davis, Representative Waxman, and members of the committee. I am Stewart Simonson, Assistant HHS Secretary for Public Health Emergency Preparedness. I appreciate the opportunity to share with you information on the Department's progress in implementing the Project BioShield Act of 2004 and our coordination with our colleagues at the Department of Homeland Security.

The events of September and October 2001 made it very clear that terrorism is a serious threat to our Nation and the world. The Bush administration and Congress responded forcefully to this threat by strengthening our medical and public health capacities to protect our citizens from future attacks. To encourage the development of new medical countermeasures against threat agents and to speed their delivery, President Bush in his 2003 State of the Union Address proposed, and Congress subsequently enacted, Project BioShield.

The $5.6 billion, 10 year special reserve fund was created to assure developers of medical countermeasures that funds would be available for the Government to purchase critical products. Since enactment, my office has moved aggressively to fill immediate gaps in our countermeasure armamentarium. A genuine sense of urgency informs all of our homeland security work at HHS.

But it is important to note that successful development and the manufacturing of safe and effective countermeasures requires an investment of both money and time. No matter how hard we try, some steps in the process cannot be rushed.

There is a complex spectrum of efforts needed along the research and development pipeline to produce a usable medical product. Defining specifications for needed countermeasures often reveals few if any candidates in the pipeline. Today, we have been fortunate that some of our highest priority needs for medical countermeasures could be addressed using the available advanced development products already in the pipeline.

However, research and development efforts, even when robustly funded, often take years before the concept is mature enough for advanced development. It is only when a product has reached the advanced development stage that Project BioShield provides a meaningful incentive for manufacturers to take the product the rest of the way.

In determining the requirements and evaluating options for medical countermeasure acquisitions, the focal point for the U.S. Government interagency effort is the Weapons of Mass Destruction Countermeasure Subcommittee. HHS, along with representatives from the Department of Homeland Security, the Department of Defense, chair of the WMD Subcommittee, and stakeholders from throughout the U.S. Government are represented on its working groups.

In setting priorities for medical countermeasure acquisition under Project BioShield, the WMD Subcommittee considers a number of factors: the credibility and immediacy of specific threats are driving factors and are informed by material threat assessments conducted by DHS. My colleague, Dr. John Vitko, here today, representing DHS, can provide insight into the assessment process.

We also consider the current and projected availability of appropriate medical countermeasures, as well as the target population for which the countermeasure would be used. In addition, logistical issues are considered, such as the feasibility of deployment in a public health emergency, shelf life and storage, and maintenance requirements.

Project BioShield requires a number of findings by the Secretaries of Homeland Security and HHS prior to an acquisition commencing. These findings include three determinations: first, that there is a material threat against the U.S. population sufficient to affect national security; second, that medical countermeasures are necessary to protect the public health from that material threat; and third, that acquiring a specific quantity of a particular medical countermeasure using the special reserve fund as appropriate.

These determinations are followed by a joint recommendation for an acquisition that is presented to the White House by the two Secretaries. If approved, Congress is notified, HHS executes the acquisition program. The process that I have outlined for you has been successfully implemented three times since the enactment of Project BioShield nearly a year ago.

HHS has completed contract awards for acquisitions of the next generation recombinant protective antigen anthrax vaccine, the current generation licensed anthrax vaccine and the pediatric formulation of potassium iodide. Additionally, the acquisition process is in the final stages for several other needed medical countermeasures, including anthrax therapeutics, botulinum antitoxin and a next generation smallpox vaccine.

This robust interagency process mines the expertise of subject matter experts in the scientific and intelligence community to define requirements for medical countermeasures and enables policymakers to identify and evaluate acquisition options to address immediate and future needs.

In closing, let me say that HHS has a clear mandate from President Bush and Congress to lead the charge in countermeasure development. We have already made important strides to address the public health needs of the Nation, but more needs to be done.

Chairman Davis, I look forward to working with you and Congressman Waxman and the rest of the committee to address the challenges of CBRN preparedness and its impact on public health. I would be glad to answer any questions.

[The prepared statement of Mr. Simonson follows:]

Testimony
Before the Committee on Government Reform
United States House of Representatives

The Role of HHS in the Development and Acquisition of Medical Countermeasures Under Project BioShield

Statement of
Stewart Simonson
Assistant Secretary
Office of Public Health Emergency Preparedness
U.S. Department of Health and Human Services

For Release on Delivery
Expected at 10:00 a.m.
Thursday, July 14, 2005

Good morning, Chairman Davis, Vice-Chairman Shays, Representative Waxman and Committee members. I am Stewart Simonson, Assistant Secretary for Public Health Emergency Preparedness, Department of Health and Human Services (HHS). I appreciate the opportunity to share with you information on the Department's progress on implementing the Project BioShield Act of 2004 ("Project BioShield") and our close coordination with colleagues in the Department of Homeland Security. Project BioShield is a vital component of our strategy to protect the Nation from threats posed from chemical, biological, radiological and nuclear (CBRN) threats. Defending against such threats is a top priority for the Bush Administration and having an appropriate armamentarium of medical countermeasures is a critical element of the response and recovery component of the President's "21st Century Strategy for Biodefense." The acquisition and ready availability of medical countermeasures, such as antibiotics, antivirals, monoclonal and polyclonal antibodies against infectious threats, therapies for chemical and radiation-induced illnesses, and vaccines to protect against exposure from biological agents are essential to our Nation's preparedness and response capabilities.

Protecting Americans

The events of September and October 2001 made it very clear that terrorism- indeed bioterrorism- is a serious threat to our Nation and the world. The Bush Administration and Congress responded forcefully to this threat by providing funding to strengthen our medical and public health capacities to protect our citizens from future attacks. Specifically, substantial increases in funding for research, development and acquisition of medical countermeasures against biological threats were directed to the National Institutes of Health (NIH) and the Centers for Disease Control and Prevention's Strategic National Stockpile (SNS or "the Stockpile"). To further encourage the development of new medical countermeasures against chemical, biological, radiological and nuclear agents and to speed their delivery and use should there be an attack, President Bush, in his 2003 State of the Union address proposed and Congress subsequently enacted Project BioShield. The Special Reserve Fund, appropriated with $5.6 billion was created to assure developers of medical countermeasures that funds would be available to purchase these critical products for use to protect our citizens.

HHS Research Efforts to Respond to CBRN Threats

Dr. Anthony Fauci, the Director of the National Institute of Allergy and Infectious Diseases (NIAID), a component of the NIH, will be testifying here today regarding the role of his institute in research and development of needed medical countermeasures for CBRN threats. NIAID is leading the Federal research enterprise in this area and Dr. Fauci will detail the Institute's efforts. I will focus my testimony on the efforts at HHS to lead the acquisition of medical countermeasures for the SNS.

The Strategic National Stockpile Today

The wake-up call that we received in the fall of 2001 highlighted the gaps in our medical countermeasure armamentarium and we immediately sought to address them. Although much remains to be done, we have made significant progress in building our Strategic National Stockpile from that time to what we have on-hand today. For example, our smallpox vaccine stockpile has grown from 90,000 ready-to-use doses in 2001 to enough vaccine to protect every man, woman, and child in America. Major strides have been made in building our medical countermeasure reserve against anthrax, plague, and tularemia. We are now able to protect and treat millions of Americans in the event of an attack with one of these agents. We have taken the botulinum antitoxin program started by the Department of Defense in the early 1990s to completion and we are now building our botulinum antitoxin stockpile further. We have also built our stockpile of countermeasures to address the effects of radiation exposure with products such as Prussian Blue and diethylenetriaminepentaacetate (DTPA). These countermeasures act to block uptake or remove radioactive elements such as cesium, thallium, or americium from the body after they are ingested or inhaled. Potassium iodide, a drug that can protect the thyroid from the harmful effects of radioactive iodine, is also in the Stockpile.

The Strategic Approach to Addressing Medical Countermeasure Gaps

The initial focus of our efforts to protect the Nation was aimed largely at those threats that could do the greatest harm to the greatest number of our citizens. Among biological threat agents, smallpox and anthrax are widely recognized as having the greatest potential to cause catastrophic harm. A sense of urgency has pervaded our efforts and we have defined new ways of doing business. Our new national security environment demands accelerated product development timelines and new paradigms of interactions between industry and government with increased risk-sharing and enhanced intra-governmental collaboration.

The focal point for USG interagency efforts to prioritize and coordinate medical countermeasures acquisition programs is the Weapons of Mass Destruction Medical Countermeasures (WMDMC) Subcommittee ("WMDMC Subcommittee"). HHS, along with representatives from the Department of Homeland Security (DHS) and the Department of Defense (DoD), co-chairs the WMDMC Subcommittee and stakeholders from throughout the USG are represented on it. Because HHS is the primary federal agency responsible for the development and acquisition of priority medical countermeasures, we have a major leadership role in the WMDMC Subcommittee.

The cornerstone of any sound acquisition program is the determination and prioritization of requirements and this is a primary activity of the WMDMC Subcommittee. In setting priorities for medical countermeasure acquisition under Project BioShield, the WMDMC Subcommittee considers a number of factors. The credibility and immediacy of the specific threats are driving factors and are informed by Material Threat Assessments (MTAs) conducted by the DHS. Dr. John Vitko, here today representing DHS, will provide insight into these efforts.

Other factors include an evaluation of the availability of appropriate countermeasures, both current and projected, and the target population for which the medical countermeasure would be used. In addition, logistical issues are considered such as the feasibility of deployment in a public health emergency, shelf life, and the storage and maintenance requirements. Project BioShield also requires a number of findings by the Secretaries of Homeland Security and HHS prior to an acquisition commencing. These findings include:

- Determination of material threat against the US population sufficient to affect national security. This determination is made by the Secretary of Homeland Security.
- Determination that countermeasures are necessary to protect public health. This determination is made by the Secretary of HHS.
- Determination of the appropriateness of funding acquisition of the countermeasure with the Special Reserve Fund (SRF). This determination is made by the Secretary of HHS.

Once these determinations are made, a joint recommendation for the acquisition is presented to the White House by the two Secretaries. If approved, Congress is notified and HHS executes the acquisition program.

The process that I have outlined for you has been successfully implemented three times since the enactment of Project BioShield less than one year ago. HHS has completed contract awards for acquisitions of the next-generation recombinant protective antigen (rPA) anthrax vaccine, the current-generation licensed anthrax vaccine (Anthrax Vaccine Adsorbed, AVA), and the pediatric formulation of potassium iodide. Additionally, the acquisition process is in the final execution phases for several other needed medical countermeasures including anthrax therapeutics, botulinum antitoxin, and a next-generation smallpox vaccine.

This robust interagency process mines the expertise of subject matter experts in the scientific and intelligence communities to define requirements for medical countermeasures and enable policy makers to identify and evaluate acquisition options to address immediate and future needs.

Application of the Strategic Approach: Anthrax.

The efficiency and effectiveness of the steps used to identify, prioritize, and acquire needed medical countermeasures is best exemplified by our efforts to protect the Nation in the event of an anthrax attack. It will also illustrate intra-agency and interagency processes.

Although anthrax is not transmissible from person-to-person, an attack involving the aerosol dissemination of anthrax spores, particularly in an urban setting, is considered by public health experts to have the potential to cause catastrophic damage. The potential for large-scale population exposure following aerosol release of anthrax spores, the threat demonstrated by the anthrax letters, and our knowledge that anthrax had been weaponized by state-actors, highlighted the nature of the threat. The Secretary of Homeland Security determined that anthrax posed a material threat to the Nation. Because untreated inhalation anthrax is usually fatal, the Secretary of HHS identified anthrax as a significant threat to public health.

The approach to protect citizens against this threat demanded immediate, intermediate and long-term strategies and requirements. First, the existing stockpile of antibiotics in the Strategic National Stockpile was increased. Second, there is a need for a licensed vaccine to be used not only for pre-exposure protection for laboratory and other workers at known risk for anthrax, but for use along with antibiotics after an exposure which could decrease the currently recommended 60-day course of antibiotic therapy. Anthrax spores are stable in the environment and would have a profound impact if released in an urban population. Therefore, availability of a vaccine may be a critical requirement for repopulation and restoration of the functionality of any exposed area.

Due to limitations inherent in the currently available anthrax vaccine, there is consensus in the scientific community about the need to develop and acquire a next-generation anthrax vaccine using 21st century technologies An assessment of developing technologies was undertaken by HHS experts in the fall of 2001 and the decision was made that there was a sufficient scientific foundation, including a detailed understanding of the pathogenesis of anthrax and how anthrax vaccines provide protective immunity, to support the aggressive development of a next generation vaccine consisting of recombinant protective antigen (rPA). The research undertaken to develop this vaccine, spanning more than a decade, was conducted in large part by the United States Army Medical Research Institute of Infectious Diseases at Fort Detrick, Maryland.

HHS defined a three-stage development and acquisition strategy with open competition for awards at each stage. The early and advanced development programs were supported by the NIAID with contract awards in September 2002 and 2003, respectively. These were milestone-driven contracts with well-defined deliverables including the manufacture of clinical-grade vaccine, the conduct of Phase I and Phase II clinical trials, and consistency lot manufacturing of vaccine. Large-scale manufacturing capacity would be required to support the civilian requirement for this medical countermeasure, which was defined by the WMD Subcommittee to be the initial protection of up to 25 million persons. Senior officials from several Departments of the USG evaluated acquisition options to achieve this requirement and, in the fall of 2003, approved the decision to pursue this acquisition of rPA anthrax vaccine.

An evaluation of the NIAID rPA anthrax vaccine development program indicated that it was robust enough to suggest that the rPA vaccine could become a licensed product within 8 years. In March 2004, the acquisition program for this vaccine, under the direction of my office, was launched using the Special

Reserve Fund created in the FY 2004 DHS appropriations bill. Utilizing a robust technical and business evaluation process, we reviewed multiple proposals and negotiated a contract for the acquisition of 75 million doses of the vaccine (anticipating a three-dose regimen). Using a milestone and deliverables approach similar to the ACAM2000 smallpox vaccine development and acquisition program, and the rPA anthrax vaccine development contracts at NIAID, the rPA vaccine BioShield acquisition contract lays out an ambitious program for the production of this vaccine. In accordance with Project BioShield, a critical aspect of this acquisition contract is the fact that no payment for product is made until a usable product is delivered to the SNS. While awaiting delivery of the rPA anthrax vaccine to the SNS, my office awarded a contract last month for 5 million doses of the currently licensed AVA vaccine to support immediate requirements. Delivery of this product to the Stockpile began soon after contract award and over one million doses of the licensed anthrax vaccine are now in the SNS.

Application of the Strategic Approach: Other Medical Countermeasures

In an effort to fill other medical countermeasure gaps, we have made progress in contracting for products that are or will soon be delivered to the SNS.

Potassium Iodide.

In March 2005 a contract was awarded under Project BioShield for a pediatric liquid formulation of potassium iodide, a drug that helps limit risk of damage to the thyroid, from radioactive iodine. This formulation is aimed at young children who have difficulty taking pills and are at the highest risk of harmful effects from exposure to radioactive iodine. This acquisition will provide needed protection for at least 1.7 million children. Product delivery began last month and should be completed by the end of the fiscal year.

Ongoing Project BioShield activities.

In addition to the acquisition contracts that have been awarded since enactment of Project BioShield, there are several other important BioShield procurement-related activities underway. We are engaged in contract negotiations for anthrax therapies, and we are continuing to move forward on the acquisition of an antitoxin treatment for botulism.

Furthermore, HHS has moved forward with the initial stages of an acquisition program for a next generation smallpox vaccine to meet a requirement for this product that addresses the millions of U.S. citizens who have contraindications for existing smallpox vaccines. A synopsis has been announced indicating that the RFP would be released later this month. This follows the consideration of industry comments received in response to a draft RFP that was released in May. We have also sought information from industry by releasing an RFI to assess the state of development of therapeutics for acute radiation syndrome.

Finally, in anticipation of yet to be determined requirements, we actively monitor the state of the medical countermeasure pipeline-- both within and outside the government--- by evaluating USG research and development portfolios and engaging industry through the publication of Requests for Information (RFIs). For example, we have recently released three RFIs to assess the timeline to maturity of medical countermeasures to treat nerve agent exposure, acute radiation syndrome, and additional products that might be available to treat anthrax. These requests are a key tool for HHS to dialogue with industry partners and to inform the development of sound USG acquisition strategies.

Priority Setting Beyond Smallpox and Anthrax

The approach taken to rapidly expand our Nation's response capacity to meet the medical and public health impact of either a smallpox or anthrax attack demonstrate our national resolve to address these threats. However, in many ways, anthrax and smallpox represent the "low hanging fruit" for medical countermeasure research, development and acquisition and was largely made possible by a substantial research base developed by USAMRIID and NIH. There was consensus that these were our highest priorities and we had countermeasures available or relatively far along in the development pipeline to permit acquisition. Given an almost endless list of potential threats with finite resources to address them, prioritization is essential to focus our efforts. We rely heavily upon our interagency partner, the Department of Homeland Security, to provide us with a prioritized list of threats along with material threat assessments that will include reasonable estimates of population exposure. This information is critical for future strategic decision making regarding how best to focus our National efforts in countermeasure development and acquisition, including whether in the short-term, the so-called "one-bug, one-drug" approach should continue while simultaneously investing in more broad-spectrum prevention and treatment approaches for the longer term.

Novel and Emerging Threats

The initial efforts for medical countermeasure development and acquisition have been rightfully focused on those threat agents known to have the potential to inflict catastrophic harm on our Nation. In addition, HHS and NIH are investing in efforts to address threat agents that we might face in the future, including engineered threats.

As is also the case for the known threat agents, we are dependent upon our colleagues at DHS to identify and prioritize these threats. One of the most recognized potential engineered threats is antibiotic-resistant anthrax, and the HHS, NIH and the U.S. Food and Drug Administration (FDA) accomplishments to date in facilitating the development and acquisition of anthrax vaccines and therapeutic antitoxins have made an important impact on reducing our vulnerabilities in this area. In addition, NIH has made a robust investment in the development of novel antimicrobial agents and in addressing all aspects of antibiotic resistance. For example, investments have been made in the development of antibacterial agents that could potentially be useful against a broad spectrum of species and a wide range of drug resistance mechanisms.

Finally, NIH is working with DoD to leverage medical countermeasure programs and resources of mutual interest.

Challenges to Rapidly Expanding the Strategic National Stockpile

Although defining priorities and quantifying the size of the threat to the population are the key steps to focus our efforts, we must be mindful of the realities of the spectrum of efforts needed along the research and development pipeline to produce a useable medical countermeasure. The process of defining required specifications for a countermeasure often reveals few, if any, candidates in the pipeline. Basic research and early development efforts, even when robustly funded, often take years before a concept is mature enough for advanced development. The development of medical products —whether for cancer, influenza, or anthrax – is a complex, lengthy, and expensive process. Ultimate licensure, approval or clearance from FDA requires the rigorous accumulation of sufficient data in humans and animals to establish the safety and efficacy of the product for a specific use and the ability to consistently manufacture the product to meet the appropriate standards. It is important to note that a unique aspect of the pathway for medical countermeasures is the need to establish efficacy either using surrogate markers (such as the human immune response) or, using appropriate animal models, under the "Animal Rule" (*Federal Register* 67:37988-37998, 2002) because demonstration of efficacy against the actual diseases in humans is most often not feasible either because the disease does not occur naturally or for the obvious ethical reasons that prevent exposing humans to the threat agent. The USG is working to provide support for the developers of priority medical countermeasures through the research and development phases, and, when a product has reached the advanced development stage Project BioShield provides an important incentive for manufacturers to take the product the rest of the way through the pipeline. And, as I have outlined here today, in the less than eleven months since Project BioShield was enacted, the incentive has expedited final development of several products for the Stockpile.

Conclusion

In closing, I must emphasize that the number of threat agents against which we could guard ourselves is endless and new and emerging threats introduced by nature or man will present continuing challenges. Although we cannot be prepared for every threat, we have the ability to create a strategic approach to identifying and combating the greatest threats. HHS and its agencies including NIH, CDC, and FDA, have a clear mandate from President Bush and Congress to lead the charge in this arena. We have already made important strides and will continue to work to address the obstacles identified. Mr. Chairman, I look forward to working with you and members of the Committee to address the challenges of bioterrorism preparedness and its impact on public health.

I will be happy to answer any questions you may have.

Chairman TOM DAVIS. Thank you, Mr. Simonson.
Dr. Fauci, thanks for being with us.

STATEMENT OF ANTHONY FAUCI, M.D.

Dr. FAUCI. Mr. Chairman, members of the committee, thank you for giving me the opportunity to discuss with you this morning the role of the NIH research enterprise in providing the basic and applied research for the development of countermeasures, some of which may ultimately go into the procurement process of BioShield; in addition, to mention to you some of the advantages that we have now for the ability to expedite our research through some of the BioShield provisions.

As shown on this first visual, you can see the covers of some of the printouts of the web-available strategic plan for biodefense research at the NIH, as well as the research agendas for the Category A and B agents. We drew this up when I testified before several committees as to the importance of having a well thought out strategic plan in the research arena, and since then, we have progress reports for the Category A as well as for the Category B and C agents.

Next slide, please. Importantly, and as mentioned in the video you showed, and in your own opening statements, we also have an important responsibility for developing countermeasures for radiological and nuclear threats. We have a strategic plan and research agenda that has just recently, within the past few weeks, been published. By the end of the year, we will have a similar plan for medical countermeasures against chemical threats.

Next visual, please. This slide summarizes some of the key achievements in the development of biodefense countermeasures, some of which are already in the procurement process, as mentioned by Mr. Simonson, some of which are in the queue for that, and others may become eligible should the material threat assessment indicate that this is the case. Importantly, with regard to smallpox, we now have, as mentioned, 300 million doses in our Strategic National Stockpile, and research is now on one of the components which is much less toxic, in the sense of less adverse events. That is modified vaccinia Ankara, in addition to anti-viral drugs.

With regard to anthrax, there is the recombinant protective antigen as well as research on antitoxins, botulism vaccine, research and development, as well as a variety of monoclonal antibodies and polyclonal antibodies against a variety of the subtypes of botulism toxin. And finally Ebola, we have conducted the first human vaccine trial for the development of an Ebola vaccine.

Next slide, please. With regard to the authorities that we now have to expedite research, we have been able to hire several high level members of our team now, particularly those who have experience in advanced development, which was one of the gaps we had, since we generally do not push products all the way through to advanced development. We expected the hiring of these through the BioShield provisions.

In addition, we have been able to expedite the awarding of grants and contracts, such as listed on this slide, by truncating the time from generally about 18 months to now between 6 and 8 months, shown here for therapeutics, antibodies protecting against botulism, as well as vaccine candidates against one type of botulism toxin.

Next slide, please. In the future, we will continue to use these BioShield authorities, some of which relate to the points you made in your statement, such as protecting the immune system against radiation by a number of protectants, as well as chelating agents, as shown in bullet No. 2, in addition to developing a variety of assays for other therapeutics.

On this final slide, it is a busy slide, and I know it is difficult to read. But the effect I want to bring up to you is that there are a number of candidates for biodefense countermeasures that are in the pipeline. What I have shown here is that if you look at the left of the slide, which is the purple bars indicating the research that we do, and if you go to the right, the orange boxes are what I would call BioShield eligible, not necessarily that it will be procured for BioShield, but that it would be advanced enough that there could be a procurement contract.

So what we generally do is the research and usually the NIH's role is to not push so far to the right in advance development.

Chairman TOM DAVIS. I hate to interrupt. Are any of these applicable to a nuclear attack?

Dr. FAUCI. Right now, the ones that we have there on this particular one are not, because we have, the nuclear component of it is still very much in what is already in the stockpile and the research is to get those licensed for the use for the civilian population. So we have a number of things in the stockpile.

The critical issue is that we are much more on the research side of new countermeasures for radio protectants, as well as for stem cell and other immune reconstitution. The reason they are not up there, Mr. Chairman, is that they haven't yet gotten to the research level to get there. We have dealings now, interactions with industry and we are trying to partner in the development of some products that have already been developed that could go into there. But there is none right there on that slide that show for nuclear.

But importantly, what we need to do is the greater partnership that you alluded to in your statement with industry to push these products through the advanced development. There has been referral to this in the situation where there are some gaps there. These are gaps that we are aware of and that we really need to fill. The basic research we do, and we can do well. The critical issue is how we get the push that we give from the research side to meet the pull that we can get from the BioShield side in order to get those products to be in our national stockpile ultimately for the protection of our Nation.

Thank you, Mr. Chairman. I would be happy to answer questions during the question period.

[The prepared statement of Dr. Fauci follows:]

Testimony
Before the Committee on Government Reform
United States House of Representatives

NIH Implementation of Project BioShield in the Research and Development of Defense Countermeasures

Statement of

Anthony S. Fauci, M.D.

Director
National Institute of Allergy and Infectious Diseases
National Institutes of Health
U.S. Department of Health and Human Services

For Release on Delivery
Expected at 10:00AM
Thursday, July 14, 2005

Introduction

Mr. Chairman and Members of the Committee, thank you for the opportunity to speak with you today concerning the role of the National Institutes of Health (NIH) in implementing the Project BioShield Act of 2004 (Public Law 108-276). This critical legislation, signed in to law by President Bush in July 2004, provided the Department of Health and Human Services (DHHS) with new authorities to develop and procure medical countermeasures that will protect the Nation in the event of a terrorist attack with a biological, chemical, nuclear, or radiological agent or device. The National Institute of Allergy and Infectious Diseases (NIAID) is the lead NIH Institute for infectious diseases research, including research and development of countermeasures against potential agents of bioterrorism. In addition, the NIAID coordinates NIH research toward the development of medical countermeasures against chemical, radiological and nuclear agents. Today, I will discuss with you the substantial progress that has been made in medical countermeasures research and development, and how Project BioShield has facilitated this progress. In addition, I will discuss some of the challenges that remain.

Components of Project BioShield

The Project BioShield Act of 2004 provided DHHS with several new authorities to facilitate a three-pronged program to expedite the development and deployment of medical countermeasures against biological, chemical, nuclear, and radiological agents. Project BioShield enabled NIH to expedite the research and development of critical medical countermeasures, established a secure funding source at DHHS for the purchase of critical medical countermeasures, and established a Food and Drug Administration (FDA) Emergency Use Authorization for critical medical countermeasures. My testimony today will focus on the implementation of NIH's BioShield authorities.

First, Project BioShield provides NIH additional flexibility in awarding contracts, cooperative agreements, and grants for research and development of critical medical countermeasures. These new authorities allow NIH to use expedited peer review procedures to obtain an assessment of the scientific and technical merit and potential contribution to the relevant field of a grant, contract, or cooperative agreement for countermeasure research. The normal NIH review and award process averages eighteen months from initial concept clearance to award; the BioShield mechanism significantly shortens this timeframe to six to eight months.

Thus far, NIAID has used Project BioShield authorities to award $29 million in grants and contracts. The activities supported by these awards will advance development of countermeasures toward possible future procurement with Project BioShield funds. These initiatives also follow recommendations in the NIAID Biodefense Research Agenda. Twelve grants have been awarded to support research and development of therapeutics directed against the CDC Category A agents that cause anthrax, smallpox, tularemia, plague, botulism, and viral hemorrhagic fevers. These grants have the potential for making a broad impact in developing therapies against the most serious agents of bioterrorism. Additionally, a contract for the development and production of monoclonal antibodies against botulinum toxin type A and a contract for the production of a recombinant vaccine candidate against botulinum toxin type E have been awarded using BioShield authorities. With each of these awards, the science already had progressed sufficiently so that NIAID is now able to undertake specific developmental activities toward possible procurement.

NIAID also has solicited applications for grants and contracts to support research on medical countermeasures against radiological or nuclear terrorist attacks, including countermeasures to protect the immune system against radiation and improved treatments for the elimination of internal radionuclide contamination that can be given by mouth rather than intravenously.

The BioShield Act also provides NIH with streamlined personnel authority. This authority allows NIH to hire individuals to fill key positions related to product development more quickly than traditional hiring processes. To date, NIAID has used Project BioShield authorities to hire two highly qualified individuals with significant product development expertise. NIAID has appointed Dr. Michael Kurilla to the dual positions of NIAID Associate Director for Biodefense Product Development and Director of the Office of Biodefense Research Affairs in the Division of Microbiology and Infectious Diseases; Dr. Bert W. Maidment, Jr. to the position of Associate Director for Product Development in the Division of Allergy, Immunology, and Transplantation; and Dr. Richard Hatchett to the position of Associate Director for Radiation Countermeasures Research and Emergency Preparedness, in the Division of Allergy, Immunology, and Transplantation,.

Project BioShield also provides NIH with additional authority for the construction of research facilities. Since the law was enacted, NIAID has used this authority to solicit applications for grants for construction of four to five additional Regional Biocontainment Laboratories (RBLs), which will support biomedical research on the NIAID Category A, B and C priority pathogens and emerging infectious diseases. These RBLs will join two National Biocontainment Laboratories (NBLs) and nine additional RBLs, the construction of which was authorized and funded in fiscal year 2003, to conduct research, train investigators, and to assist National, State and local public health efforts in the event of a deliberately released (bioterrorism) or naturally occurring infectious disease emergency.

As noted above, Project BioShield provides DHHS with the authority and funding to procure promising countermeasures for the Strategic National Stockpile (SNS), which is administered by the Centers for Disease Control and Prevention (CDC). It also provides the authority to grant emergency authorization for the use of unapproved countermeasures if, among other things, the FDA

Commissioner determines that there is no adequate approved alternative available.

Certain pharmaceutical and biotechnology companies have proven to be willing and eager to help in the development of biodefense countermeasures, but they need a reasonable assurance that a market for these products will in fact exist should they invest the resources necessary to fully develop them. To help provide these incentives, Project BioShield established a Special Reserve Fund for the purchase of biodefense countermeasures for the SNS for use in an emergency. Through these authorities, Project BioShield has given us new ways to both "push" and "pull" science toward needed countermeasures; NIH-supported basic research provides the "push", and guaranteed funding for procurement of these countermeasures provides the "pull" needed to attract industry.

Advanced Development

NIH historically has supported research that generates new knowledge about disease and has worked to translate these findings into vaccines, therapeutics, and diagnostics that protect public health. Working in close collaboration with industry, NIAID supported the advanced development of a next-generation anthrax vaccine that has since been procured by DHHS using BioShield funds. NIAID also is supporting trials of a next-generation smallpox vaccine, which would be eligible for future BioShield procurement.

NIAID played a major role in the rapid development of the next-generation anthrax vaccine known as recombinant protective antigen, or rPA. The applied research and advanced development of rPA were supported by the NIAID with contracts awarded in September 2002 and 2003, respectively. These were milestone-driven contracts with well-defined goals including the manufacture of clinical-grade vaccine, the conduct of Phase I and Phase II clinical trials, and consistency lot manufacturing of vaccine. Clinical trials to evaluate rPA are currently underway. To date, the immune responses elicited in humans are similar to those elicited in animal studies, which have demonstrated that the rPA vaccine protected animals against aerosol challenge with anthrax spores. Last November, DHHS awarded a contract for the acquisition of 75 million doses of rPA vaccine to be held in the SNS. NIAID's rPA product development initiatives were instrumental in making the SNS initiative possible.

NIAID-supported researchers also are developing and testing a new smallpox vaccine, modified vaccinia Ankara (MVA), which causes fewer side effects than the traditional "Dryvax" vaccine because it does not replicate effectively in human cells. NIAID has supported the advanced development of MVA through milestone-driven contract awards in 2003 and 2004. Early clinical trials in small numbers of human volunteers have demonstrated the MVA vaccine to be safe and immunogenic, and animal studies by the developers are confirming earlier studies by NIAID and Department of Defense (DoD) scientists showing that MVA protects monkeys and mice from smallpox-like viruses. Based on these results and the demonstration of the feasibility of large-scale manufacturing capacity, DHHS has moved forward with the initial stages of an MVA acquisition program.

NIAID's support for the advanced development of the rPA and MVA vaccines was a unique commitment that was begun prior to the BioShield legislation. The advanced development of these two vaccines was enabled by a substantial research base developed by the DoD and NIAID.

Biodefense Research Priorities

The NIH biodefense research agenda was developed through a comprehensive and systematic strategic planning process. In February 2002, NIH convened the Blue Ribbon Panel on Bioterrorism and Its Implications for Biomedical Research, with membership composed of distinguished researchers from academic centers, private industry, government civilian agencies, and the military. Three key documents were developed based on this panel's advice and on extensive discussions with other Federal agencies: the *NIAID Strategic Plan for Biodefense Research*, the *NIAID Research Agenda for CDC Category A Agents*, and the *NIAID Research Agenda for CDC Category B and C Agents* (agents whose biological properties make them more difficult to deploy or less likely to cause widespread harm than a Category A agent). It is important to note that NIAID maintains an NIAID list of Category A, B and C Priority Pathogens which closely follows the CDC list of Category A, B and C Biological Diseases/Agents. The

NIAID list highlights specific pathogens identified as priorities for additional research efforts as part of the NIAID biodefense research agenda. The Strategic Plan provides a blueprint for the conduct of basic research on microbes and host immune defenses, as well as targeted, milestone-driven development of drugs, vaccines, diagnostics and other interventions that would be needed in the event of a bioterror attack. The two biodefense research agendas describe short-term, intermediate, and long-term goals for research on the wide variety of agents that could be used to conduct such an attack.

We developed the *Strategic Plan* and the two research agendas based on an overall threat assessment formulated by CDC in close cooperation with the intelligence community. Category A agents are the most dangerous microbes and toxins; these agents cause diseases that include anthrax, smallpox, plague, botulism, tularemia, and hemorrhagic fevers. These agents were given the highest priority because they: (a) are relatively easily disseminated or transmitted from person to person; (b) result in high mortality rates with the potential for major public health impact; (c) would likely cause significant social disruption; and (d) require special action for public health preparedness. Category B agents are in the second tier of priority. They are agents that: (a) are moderately easy to disseminate, (b) result in moderate morbidity and low mortality, and (c) require specific enhancements of national diagnostic capacity and disease surveillance systems. Category C Agents have the next highest priority. They include emerging pathogens that could be engineered for mass dissemination in the future because of their availability, ease of production and dissemination, and potential for high rates of morbidity and mortality and major health impact.

NIAID also recently completed a Strategic Plan to accelerate the development and deployment of new medical countermeasures against ionizing radiation for the civilian population, and DHHS has tasked NIAID with drafting a strategic plan and research agenda to guide development of medical countermeasures against chemical threats. Input from several expert panels will be incorporated into a Strategic Plan and Research Agenda for countermeasure research against the leading chemical threats of concern to public health. Both the plan and agenda are expected to be complete by the end of this calendar year. I would note that efforts are underway, in partnership with other research institutes of the NIH and the DoD, to address medical countermeasures against chemical threats.

To obtain information about new threats that may arise, DHHS relies heavily on the Department of Homeland Security (DHS) to provide a prioritized list of threats along with Material Threat Determinations (MTDs) that will provide reasonable estimates of population exposure. DHS has issued MTDs for attacks with the agents that cause anthrax and smallpox, attacks with botulinum toxin, and nuclear and radiological attacks; MTDs against additional agents are underway. This information is critical for strategic decision-making on how best to focus our future efforts in countermeasure development. Because new infectious diseases emerge naturally on a regular basis, NIH has considerable experience in rapidly mobilizing research resources to confront new infectious disease threats. This experience serves us well when we are called upon to adjust our research priorities in response to new intelligence information. In addition, this information is necessary to fully engage the pharmaceutical and biotechnology industries in countermeasures development; without MTDs, industry has no way of knowing which high-priority products are being considered for procurement for the SNS.

NIAID's long experience with infectious disease research allowed us to take on a greatly expanded role in civilian biodefense after the terrorist attacks in the fall of 2001, and I am confident that we are making good progress. Project BioShield has provided us with some of the tools necessary to accelerate and expand the basic and applied research, advanced development, and ultimate procurement of safe and effective vaccines, therapeutics, and diagnostics against biological, chemical, nuclear, and radiological agents. We have already begun using these tools to support important research for our nation's defense. I look forward to working with you, Mr. Chairman, and with this Committee, to continue to address the challenges involved in the research and development of biodefense countermeasures.

I appreciate this opportunity to testify before you today, and I would be pleased to answer any questions that you may have.

NIH Implementation of Project BioShield in the Research and Development of Biodefense Countermeasures

U.S. House of Representatives Committee on Government Reform

Dr. Anthony S. Fauci, M.D.
Director
National Institute of Allergy and Infectious Diseases
National Institutes of Health
Department of Health and Human Services
July 14, 2005

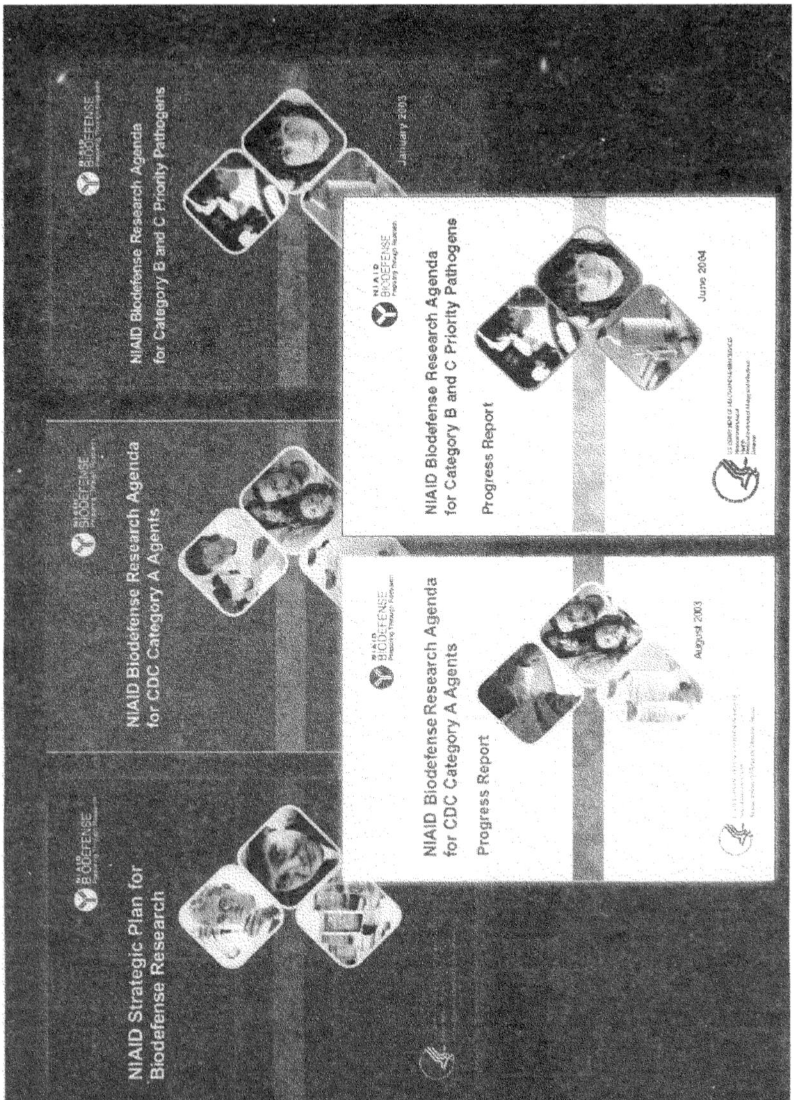
NIAID BIODEFENSE
NIAID Strategic Plan for Biodefense Research
NIAID BIODEFENSE
NIAID Biodefense Research Agenda for CDC Category A Agents
NIAID BIODEFENSE
NIAID Biodefense Research Agenda for Category B and C Priority Pathogens
January 2003
NIAID BIODEFENSE
NIAID Biodefense Research Agenda for CDC Category A Agents
Progress Report
August 2003
NIAID BIODEFENSE
NIAID Biodefense Research Agenda for Category B and C Priority Pathogens
Progress Report
June 2004

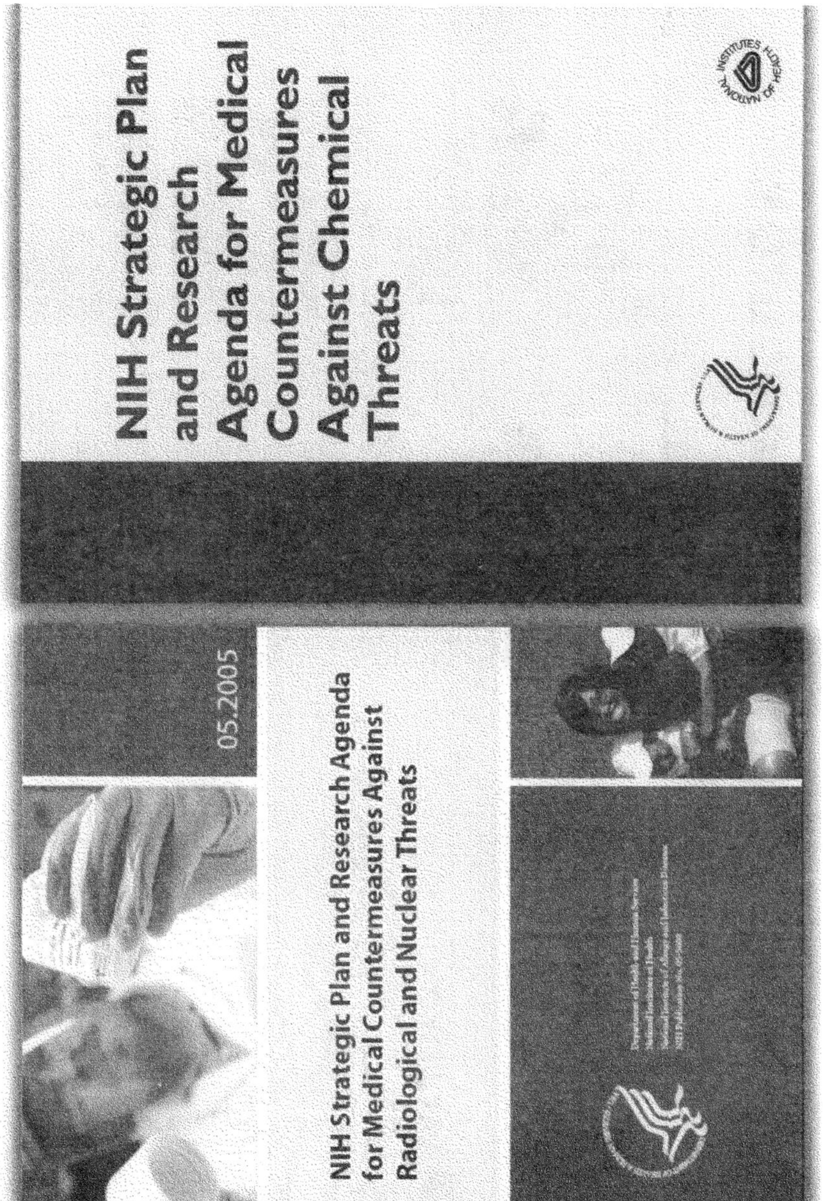
NIH Strategic Plan and Research Agenda for Medical Countermeasures Against Chemical Threats
05.2005
NIH Strategic Plan and Research Agenda for Medical Countermeasures Against Radiological and Nuclear Threats

Biodefense Countermeasures: Key Achievements

- Smallpox
  - Dryvax; MVA; antiviral drugs

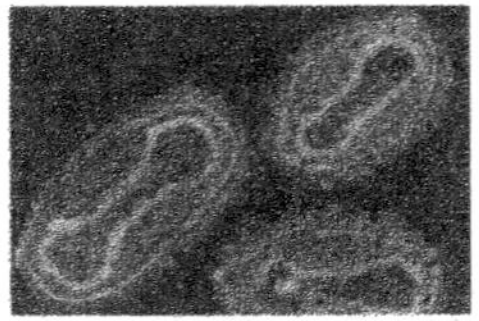

- Anthrax
  - rPA; antitoxins

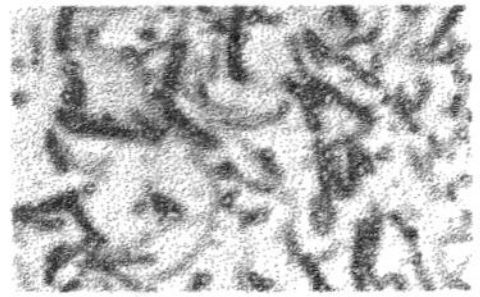

- Botulinum
  - Vaccine; antitoxins

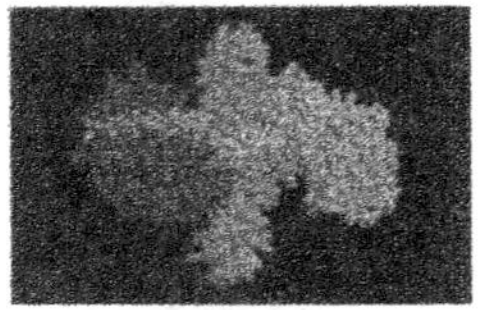

- Ebola
  - First human vaccine trials

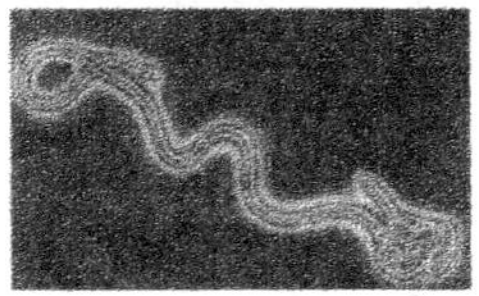

Recent NIH Awards Using BioShield Authorities

Awards ($29M):

- Therapeutics for CDC Category A Agents
- Development and Production of Antibodies that Protect Against Botulinum Toxin Type A
- Production of a Vaccine Candidate Against Botulinum Toxin Type E

Future NIH Awards Using BioShield Authorities

Future Awards:

- Protecting the Immune System Against Radiation: BioShield Accelerated Product Development (FY 2005; $4M)
- Development of Improved DTPA for Radionuclide Chelation (FY 2005; $6M)
- Assays for Influenza Therapeutics (FY 2006; $10M)

Budgeted Milestones for Development of BioShield Priority Countermeasures

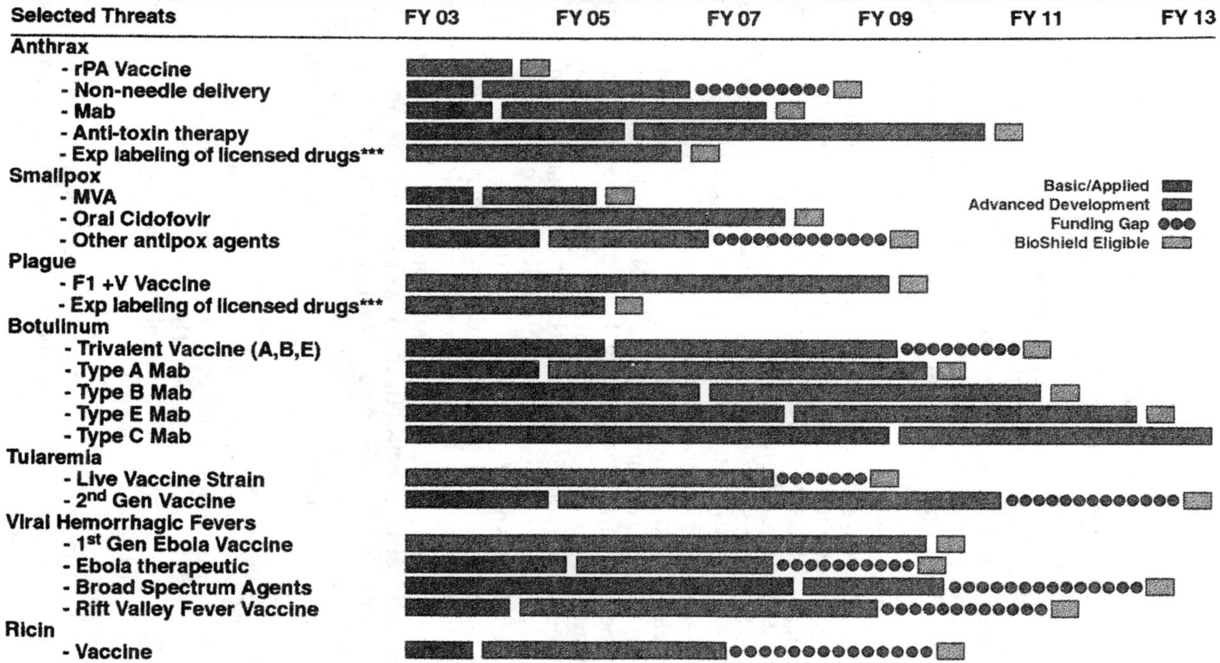

*** Previously licensed for other indications

Chairman TOM DAVIS. Thank you.
Dr. Vitko.

STATEMENT OF JOHN VITKO, JR.

Dr. VITKO. Good afternoon, Congressman Davis, Congressman Waxman and distinguished members of the committee. I am pleased to appear before you today to discuss the Department of Homeland Security's efforts in Project BioShield implementation, including the development of threat and risk assessments that help inform and priorities BioShield research, development and procurement, as well as our close coordination with the Department of Health and Human Services throughout the process.

I will begin with a description of coordination between DHS and HHS on near-term implementation of BioShield and then move on to three major activities to support and guide future BioShield acquisitions: risk assessments across a broad set of biological agents, a strategy for addressing the engineered threat, and scientific research to reduce key uncertainties in these risk assessments.

The Project BioShield Act of 2004 charges the Secretary of Homeland Security with the responsibility to determine which biological, chemical, radiological and nuclear threats constitute a material threat to our Nation's security. To fulfill this responsibility, the DHS Science and Technology Directorate, in partnership with our Information Analysis and Infrastructure Protection Directorate, has been conducting formal threat assessments of the agents of greatest concern to establish plausible high consequence scenarios.

These assessments combine intelligence information with technical assessments of the feasibility of a terrorist to produce and disseminate the agent, to provide an indication of the number of exposed individuals, the geographical extent of the exposure and other collateral effects. If these consequences are of such a magnitude to be of significant concern to our national security or public health, the Secretary of DHS then issues a formal material threat determination to the Secretary of HHS, which initiates the BioShield process.

HHS, assisted by the Interagency Weapons of Mass Destruction Medical Countermeasures Subcommittee, then determines the need for and requirements of any new medical countermeasures. Any recommendations issued for the acquisition of a specific countermeasure are evaluated through an interagency process and form the basis of the U.S. Government requirements.

After approval of these requirements by the Office of Management and Budget, HHS issues a request for proposals and implements and manages the subsequent acquisition process through the delivery of the countermeasures to the Strategic National Stockpile. As described above, the normal process is to have an in-depth threat and risk assessment precede the material threat determinations.

However, four threats were recognized to be of such urgency that the Secretary of DHS issued material threat determinations for them soon after the enactment of BioShield legislation and concurrently initiated in-depth assessments of plausible high consequence scenarios to better inform procurement requirements. These four threats are anthrax, smallpox, botulinum toxin and radiological and nuclear devices.

Subsequently, full assessments have been performed on anthrax and botulinum toxin and radiological devices and a special study conducted on fissile materials, i.e., nuclear weapons. HHS has moved out promptly in addressing these threats with contracts in place for first and second generation anthrax vaccines and a pediatric formulation of potassium iodide. HHS is also in the acquisition process for botulinum toxin, anthrax therapeutics and the next generation of smallpox vaccines and has issued a number of requests for information for other medical countermeasures.

We at DHS are currently addressing the next tier of threats. Assessments are nearly complete for plague, tularemia and chemical nerve agents. An assessment of viral hemorrhagic fevers will be completed this fiscal year. Based on the outcomes of these assessments, the Secretary of DHS may issue additional material threat determinations.

The threat assessments and procurement actions discussed above focus on those CBRN agents widely agreed to be of greatest concern since the near-term BioShield processes. We are also conducting three key activities to guide future rounds of BioShield acquisitions. As part of our responsibilities under the President's strategy for biodefense for the 21st century, we are conducting a formal risk assessment across a broad range of biological threats, including all Category A and B agents from the Centers for Disease Control and Prevention threat list, some Category C agents and a number of potential engineered threats.

These risk assessments factor in technical feasibility producing and disseminating the threat, the vulnerability of different portions of our society to those threats, and the resulting consequences of any such attack. Looking still further into the future, we have partnered with HHS and others in formulating and implementing a strategy for anticipating and responding to engineered threats. Together, we have developed an informed estimate of the types of emerging threats that might be within the ability of a terrorist organization to develop over the near, mid and longer terms, and have laid out a strategy for addressing them.

Realizing that there are still large uncertainties, sometimes factors of 10 to 100, in some of the key parameters underlying these threat and risk assessments, we have established a National Biodefense Analysis and Countermeasures Center [NBACC], to conduct the laboratory experiments needed to reduce these uncertainties. Pending the completion of construction of the associated facility on the Fort Detrick campus in 2008, interim capabilities have been established with other Government and private laboratories to begin this vital work.

In summary, DHS science and technology threat and risk assessments play a critical role in prioritizing BioShield acquisitions. Throughout the process, we have worked closely with our colleagues at HHS to most effectively couple DHS expertise on the threat and risk with HHS expertise on human health to better protect the Nation.

This concludes my prepared statement. Mr. Chairman, Congressman Waxman, and members of the committee, I thank you for the opportunity to appear before you. I will be happy to answer any questions that you may have.

[The prepared statement of Dr. Vitko follows:]

Statement for the Record

Dr. John Vitko, Jr.
Director, Biological Countermeasures Portfolio
Science & Technology Directorate
Department of Homeland Security

Before the U.S. House of Representatives
Committee on Government Reform

July 14, 2005

INTRODUCTION

Good afternoon, Chairman Davis, Congressman Waxman, and distinguished members of the Committee. I am pleased to appear before you today to discuss the role of the Department of Homeland Security (DHS) in implementing Project BioShield and our close coordination with the Department of Health and Human Services throughout this process.

Before focusing on the Department's specific activities in support of Project Bioshield, I would like to put these activities in the broader context of the overall responsibilities and activities of the DHS Biological Countermeasures Portfolio (Bio Portfolio) which I direct. The mission of this Portfolio is to provide the understanding, technologies, and systems needed to anticipate, deter, protect against, detect, mitigate, and recover from possible biological attacks on this nation's population, agriculture or infrastructure.

In addressing this mission, DHS has a leadership role in several key areas, and a partnership role in others. Those areas in which the Science and Technology (S&T) Directorate has a significant leadership role are in:

- Providing an overall end-to-end understanding of an integrated biodefense strategy, so as to guide the Secretary and the rest of the Department in its responsibility to coordinate the nation's efforts to deter, detect, and respond to acts of biological terrorism.

- Providing scientific support to understand better both current and future biological threats and their potential impacts so as to guide the research and development of biodefense countermeasures such as vaccines, drugs, detection systems and decontamination technologies.

- Developing early warning, detection and characterization systems to permit timely response to mitigate the consequence of a biological attack.

- Conducting technical forensics to analyze and interpret materials recovered from an attack to support attribution.

- Operation of the Plum Island Animal Disease Center to support both research and development (R&D) and operational response to foreign animal diseases such as foot and mouth disease.

DHS also supports our partnering departments and agencies with their leads in other key areas of an integrated biodefense: the Department of Health and Human Services (HHS) on medical countermeasures and mass casualty response; the Department of Defense (DoD) on broad range of homeland security/homeland defense issues; the U.S. Department of Agriculture (USDA) on agriculture biosecurity; USDA and HHS on food defense; the Department of Veterans' Affairs (VA) on maintaining pharmaceutical caches (antidotes, vaccines and ventilators); the Environmental Protection Agency (EPA) on decontamination and on water safety; the Department of Justice on bioterrorism investigations; and the Intelligence Community on threat warnings.

Today I would like to focus on those aspects of our work that play a major role in BioShield implementation. I will begin with a description of the coordination between DHS and HHS on the near-term implementation of the BioShield Program and then move on to three major activities to support and guide future BioShield acquisitions: risk assessments across a broader set of biological agents; a strategy for addressing the engineered threat; and scientific research to reduce key uncertainties in these risk assessments. In the course of these discussions, I will also address the specific questions that the Committee raised in their invitation letter to this hearing.

COORDINATION BETWEEN DHS AND HHS ON NEAR-TERM IMPLEMENTATION OF THE BIOSHIELD PROGRAM

The Project BioShield Act of 2004 charges the Secretary of Homeland Security with the responsibility to determine which biological, chemical, radiological or nuclear threats constitute a Material Threat to our Nation's security. To fulfill this responsibility, the DHS Science and Technology Directorate, in partnership with our Information Analysis and Infrastructure Protection Directorate, has been conducting formal threat assessments of the agents of greatest concern to establish plausible high consequence scenarios. These assessments combine intelligence information with technical assessments of the feasibility of a terrorist to produce and disseminate the agent to provide an indication of the number of exposed individuals, the geographical extent of the exposure, and other collateral effects. If these consequences are of such a magnitude to be of significant concern to our national security or public health, the Secretary of DHS then issues a formal Material Threat Determination to the Secretary of HHS, which initiates the BioShield process. Subsequently, HHS, assisted by the interagency Weapons of Mass Destruction Medical Countermeasures subcommittee, determines the need for, and requirements of, any new medical countermeasures. Any recommendations issued for the acquisition of a specific countermeasure are evaluated through an interagency process and form the basis of the U.S. Government requirements. After approval of these requirements by the Office of Management and Budget, HHS issues a Request for Proposals and implements and manages the subsequent acquisition process through delivery of the countermeasures to the Strategic National Stockpile.

As described above, the normal process is to have an in depth threat and risk assessment precede the Material Threat Determination. However, four threats were recognized to be of such urgency, that the Secretary of DHS issued Material Threat Determinations for them soon after the enactment of BioShield legislation and concurrently initiated in depth assessments of plausible high consequence scenarios to better inform procurement requirements. These four threats are anthrax, smallpox, botulinum toxin, and radiological/nuclear devices. Subsequently, full assessments have been performed on anthrax, botulinum toxin, and radiological devices and a special study conducted on fissile materials. HHS has moved out promptly in addressing these threats, with contracts in place for first and second generation anthrax vaccines, and a pediatric formulation of potassium iodide. HHS is also in the acquisition process for botulinum antitoxin, anthrax therapeutics, and the next generation of smallpox vaccine, and has issued a number of Requests for Information (RFIs) for other medical countermeasures.

We are currently addressing the next tier of threats. Assessments are nearly complete for plague, tularemia, and chemical nerve agents, and an assessment of viral hemorrhagic fevers will be initiated in August. Based on the outcomes of these assessments, the Secretary of DHS may issue additional Material Threat Determinations.

Risk Assessments Across a Broader Range of Biological Threats

The preceding discussion dealt with threat assessments and near-term BioShield acquisitions of countermeasures against those CBRN agents widely agreed to be of greatest concern. As part of its responsibility in the President's National Biodefense Strategy, DHS is conducting a formal risk assessment of a much broader set of biological agents to help prioritize the nation's ongoing biodefense activities, including subsequent rounds of BioShield acquisitions. These risk assessments provide a systematic evaluation of the technical feasibility of a broad range of biological threats, the vulnerability of different portions of our society to those threats, and the resulting consequences of any such attacks.

The first such formal risk assessment is due in the January of 2006, with subsequent assessments due every two years. The scope, process, and timescale for this first assessment have been presented to and agreed to by the interagency Biodefense Policy Coordinating Committee co-chaired by the Homeland Security Council and the National Security Council. This assessment is addressing:

- All six category A agents from the Centers for Disease Control and Prevention (CDC) threat list;
- All 12 category B agents;
- Five representative category C agents; and
- A number of candidate drug-resistant and emerging agents.

Key outputs will include:

- A list of bio-threats prioritized by risk;
- A prioritized list of critical knowledge gaps that if closed should reduce risk assessment uncertainty and guide biodefense research and development; and
- A list of biodefense vulnerabilities that could be reduced by countermeasure development and acquisition.

This risk assessment is being conducted in partnership with the Intelligence Community, the HHS, the Department of Defense, the U.S. Department of Agriculture, the Environmental Protection Agency and others. Two advisory boards, one a Government Stakeholders Advisory Board and the other an Independent Risk Assessment Expert

Review Board (academia, industry, and government), have been established to provide input and advice.

This and subsequent risk assessments will play a critical role in informing future biodefense programs across all agencies, including BioShield acquisitions and the longer-term medical R&D leading up to such acquisitions.

A Strategy for Addressing Emerging Threats

Much of the biodefense efforts to date have focused on protecting against attacks with bioterrorism agents that can be (or used to be) found in nature. However, rapid advances in biotechnology demand that we also consider the possibility and impact of emerging or engineered agents. e.g. modifications to organisms that increase their resistance to medical countermeasure or make them more difficult to detect. The President's *Biodefense for the 21st Century* assigns the HHS the lead in anticipating such future threats. The S&T Directorate is partnering with HHS and others in formulating and implementing a strategy for anticipating and responding to such threats.

Based on intelligence information, available literature and expert judgment, we have developed an informed estimate of the types of emerging threats that might be within the ability of a terrorist organization to develop over the near (1-3 years), mid (4-10 years), and longer-terms (10 yrs). We have also examined the impact of these threats on the four pillars of the National Biodefense Policy as articulated in Homeland Security Presidential Directive (HSPD)-10: Threat Awareness, Prevention and Protection, Surveillance and Detection, and Response and Recovery.

In this analysis, four elements stand out as essential to an effective defense against emerging threats:

- Threat, vulnerability and risk assessments to prioritize these threats in terms of the difficulty of their development and deployment, as well as their potential consequences;
- Surveillance and detection capabilities to rapidly detect and characterize engineered agents in environmental and clinical samples so as to provide timely guidance in the selection of the appropriate medical countermeasure;
- An expanded range of safe and effective medical countermeasures and an infrastructure to support rapid research, development, test, and evaluation (RDT&E) of new medical countermeasures; and
- Integrated concepts of operation (CONOPS) for the identification and response to emerging threats. In addition to conducting these assessments, DHS will continue to collaborate with HHS as it leads efforts to anticipate agents and to facilitate the availability of medical countermeasures.

Scientific research to better inform these threat and risk assessments

The threat and risk assessments described above are performed with the best available information. However, there are large uncertainties, sometimes factors of ten to a hundred, in some of the key parameters and hence in the associated risks. One of the major functions of the threat and risk assessments is to identify these critical knowledge gaps, which can differ for different threat scenarios – in one case it can be the minimum amount of agent needed to infect a person; in another case it can be the time that such an agent remains viable (capable of causing an infection) in the air, food or water; and in a third it can be the effect of food processing or water treatment on the agent's viability. Conducting the laboratory experiments to close the critical knowledge gaps is a primary function of DHS's National Biodefense Analysis and Countermeasures Center (NBACC).

Congress has appropriated a total of $128M for design and construction of NBACC with the necessary biocontainment laboratory space and support infrastructure to conduct these and other experiments. NBACC will be built on the National Interagency Biodefense Campus (NIBC) at Ft. Detrick MD, where it is in close proximity to the DoD's United States Army Medical Research Institute for Infectious Diseases (USAMRIID), the NIH's Integrated Research Facility and the USDA's Foreign Disease-Weed Science Research Unit. NBACC is also collaborating with the Centers for Disease Control and Prevention to further address the critical knowledge gaps. The Record of Decision for NBACC's Final Environmental Impact Statement was signed in January 2005. Design of the facility began in March 2005, with construction scheduled to begin in FY 2006 and be complete by the fourth quarter of FY 2008.

Currently, interim capabilities for both NBACC's biological threat awareness and bioforensic analysis functions have been established with other government and private laboratories to allow vital work in these areas to occur during the NBACC facility's construction

CONCLUSION

In summary, the DHS Science and Technology Directorate's programs in threat and risk assessment play a critical role in prioritizing both near and longer-term BioShield research, development, and procurements for medical countermeasures. Throughout this process we work closely with our colleagues at HHS through a variety of interagency, bi-lateral, and informal scientist-to-scientist interactions so as to most effectively couple DHS expertise on the threat and risk with HHS expertise on human health to better protect our Nation.

This concludes my prepared statement. With the Committee's permission, I request my formal statement be submitted for the record. Mr. Chairman, Congressman Waxman, and Members of the Committee, I thank you for the opportunity to appear before you and I will be happy to answer any questions that you may have.

Chairman TOM DAVIS. Thank you very much.

Mr. Simonson, I am going to start with you. One of the chief purposes of the Project BioShield Act was to enable the Government to more rapidly acquire countermeasures against biological, chemical, radiological or nuclear agents that might be used in terrorist attacks. The administration has identified the following agents for which countermeasures are needed to protect the public health: anthrax, smallpox, botulism toxin, plague and Ebola.

Has the Department of Health and Human Services used any of the special acquisition flexibilities contained in the act, such as the enhanced simplified acquisition authority and expanded sole source authority for BioShield procurement conducted to date?

Mr. SIMONSON. No. Our view has been that we wanted to, where possible, compete in full and open competition to keep the price down for these drugs. So to date, we have not had a need to use those authorities.

Chairman TOM DAVIS. I understand that you have issued a request for information for drugs that might prove effective in treating acute radiation exposure and radiation sickness and that you have announced the intention to issue a draft RFP for this purpose by the end of the month, is that correct?

Mr. SIMONSON. Yes.

Chairman TOM DAVIS. I think there remains a concern that this process of reviewing, procurement and stockpiling effective radiological and nuclear countermeasures will drag on for several more months. Can you explain why you have chosen a draft RFP instead of an RFP?

Mr. SIMONSON. It is a way to ensure that the ultimate acquisition is done properly. We issue the draft RFP to give industry an opportunity to comment on it. I think we have seen in the past that sometimes when RFPs go out, we are asking for things that we simply can't get from industry or we are asking for them in a format that doesn't work. We have found that the draft RFP mechanism helps us from having to duplicate efforts subsequently, for example, to recall——

Chairman TOM DAVIS. But a regular RFP has to follow that, right?

Mr. SIMONSON. Oh, yes. But oftentimes the time lines are compressed, leveraging some of the draft RFP time, knowing that the——

Chairman TOM DAVIS. It reminds me of a friend of mine who was engaged to be engaged. It was one of those things. I guess it moves the process down a little bit, but you still have some——

Mr. SIMONSON. Right.

Chairman TOM DAVIS. Well, let me ask you this. Nothing currently exists in the Strategic National Stockpile for radiation protection that addresses acute radiation syndrome.

Mr. SIMONSON. There are things in the Stockpile that do. We have a number of things in the Stockpile. You mentioned potassium iodide. Our only BioShield acquisition for radiation sickness is suspension potassium iodide for children.

But in the Stockpile we have and have been building up products that are used to treat internal radiation exposure, they are called chelating agents.

Chairman TOM DAVIS. Dr. Fauci, if you want to join in on this, because we need to know this.

Mr. SIMONSON. Yes. This is called zinc and calcium DTPA. We have a drug called Prussian Blue. We have a drug called Nupogen, which is used to treat acute neutropenia, which is what follows radiation exposure. So we do have Stockpile elements that are responsive to radiation exposure.

We also have a fair amount of what are called burn and blast provisions to be used.

Chairman TOM DAVIS. But you concede it is not where you want to be?

Mr. SIMONSON. No, no, absolutely not.

Chairman TOM DAVIS. When do you anticipate actually getting this new drug developed and stockpiling that? Do you see a time line? You have this draft RFP that is coming, and you will have an RFP, and you will get the responses. Do you have any idea what the time line might be?

Mr. SIMONSON. I can't give you the exact time line.

Chairman TOM DAVIS. I understand.

Mr. SIMONSON. I will tell you that we want it sooner rather than later, as fast as possible. But I have to be very careful about entering into an acquisition, I think this committee can be sensitive to this, where we have a malfunction of the Federal acquisition regulations or something like that, we do it in a very deliberate and cautious way. I do not think it is overly cautious, however.

Chairman TOM DAVIS. How prepared would we be today if the recent anthrax incident at the D.C. Postal Service and DOD facilities had been even more widespread, or if an airborne anthrax attack from a small plane were to occur in Metropolitan Washington, requiring drugs and vaccinations for those exposed and for first responders?

Mr. SIMONSON. We are substantially better prepared than we were in October 2001. We have enormous quantities of antibiotics in the Strategic National Stockpile to treat tens of millions of people for full courses of treatment, full 60 day courses of treatment. We have, under the operation of DHS, a very reliable system for monitoring exposure, the so-called Biowatch system.

We have 5 million, as you noted, 5 million doses of the currently licensed anthrax vaccine in the Stockpile. We have an RFP, well, not an RFP, we are seeking to negotiate an option for an additional 5 million doses of that material. Then we have the contract for 75 million doses of the next generation material, recombinant protective antigen.

Chairman TOM DAVIS. Thank you.

Mr. Waxman.

Mr. WAXMAN. Thank you, Mr. Chairman.

Mr. Simonson, to prepare for pandemic influenza, the administration has purchased 5.3 million courses of the anti-viral drug Tamiflu for the National Stockpile. Is that enough?

Mr. SIMONSON. No.

Mr. WAXMAN. The administration has purchased 2 million doses of a vaccine against avian flu to have on hand to vaccinate health care workers while a pandemic vaccine is manufactured. Is this enough?

Mr. SIMONSON. It is enough for the beginning, yes. This was never meant to be a discrete and final action. This is the beginning of a program to purchase sufficient quantities of vaccine to enable us to respond to a pandemic.

I might add that we were the first to do this. Dr. Fauci can comment on this.

Mr. WAXMAN. In terms of making it available to all of our health care workers, do we have enough?

Mr. SIMONSON. No, but we don't know enough about the vaccine to say even how it would be used at this point. There are clinical studies going on in Dr. Fauci's lab which will inform that. Again, we were the first in the world to do that.

Mr. WAXMAN. Only a handful of States have the full capacity to deploy and distribute the Strategic National Stockpile. Is that enough?

Mr. SIMONSON. No.

Mr. WAXMAN. The company says it will close the only smallpox vaccine production facility in the United States if it does not get a Government contract to maintain its ability to produce the vaccine. Should this facility close down?

Mr. SIMONSON. It is news to me that they are suggesting that. We are in discussion with them now about the proper way to maintain a warm base at that facility.

Mr. WAXMAN. The company BioPort says it may be forced to close the only anthrax vaccine production facility in the United States if it does not get a Government contract to maintain its ability to produce the vaccine. Should this facility close down?

Mr. SIMONSON. Should it close down? We are not advocating for it to be closed down, obviously, and we——

Mr. WAXMAN. Would you be concerned if it did, because of the argument that they don't have a Government contract to get enough money to produce the vaccine?

Mr. SIMONSON. As I said, we have made an acquisition of what we believe our requirement is at this point, 5 million doses of AVA. We are seeking an option for an additional 5 million doses.

But as you can imagine, in our world, we hear this often: if the Government doesn't do this, if the Government doesn't do that, we will close down. Frankly, we have to be responsive to what it is that we need for the Stockpile.

Mr. WAXMAN. Two weeks ago, this committee heard testimony from Dr. Fauci and Dr. Bruce Gellin that the United States needed to purchase more courses of the anti-viral drug Tamiflu. So far the United States has purchased enough for only about 2 percent of the population, about 5 million courses of treatment.

I have learned that from the company Roche that 7 million courses of treatment are available for sale from next year's production. If we need more and more is for sale, why haven't we ordered more?

Mr. SIMONSON. Well, I should say that we are in discussion with Roche about their production capability and what they can provide us. They are aware of our preliminary plans.

However, it is worth pointing out that much like with the vaccine, we were well ahead of others in buying anti-virals. Other countries are often cited as having these enormous anti-viral stockpiles. Few have more than we have right now. We were——

Mr. WAXMAN. But if we have only for 2 percent of the population, that doesn't sound right. Would you support the United States purchasing all 7 million available courses of the treatment?

Mr. SIMONSON. We are interested in more Tamiflu.

Mr. WAXMAN. OK. Has the availability of funds in any way hindered your ability to contract for doses of Tamiflu that you believe are important to protect the American people?

Mr. SIMONSON. I am not aware of a funding constraint at this point, but I am not a budgetary person.

Mr. WAXMAN. If you have to purchase more Tamiflu and they want a certain amount of money and you don't have it, isn't that a problem?

Mr. SIMONSON. It is not clear to me that we don't have it.

Mr. WAXMAN. Oh. OK. Well, we will be interested in hearing more about that.

The purpose of BioShield is to encourage the development of new and innovative countermeasures against serious public health threats. The White House, for example, has said that the program is intended to create and procure countermeasures that are modern, new and next generation. Yet as I mentioned in my opening statement, HHS recently took $120 million in BioShield funds to purchase 5 million doses of anthrax vaccine that was licensed in 1970. Do you think that was a good idea, or should we be using it for future innovation?

Mr. SIMONSON. I think it was a very good idea. And it was contemplated in the statute. The statute says, a security countermeasure without a commercial market, other than as a security countermeasure. That describes the BioPort vaccine. And as we have, I think agreed, it is an important vaccine to have in the Stockpile.

Mr. WAXMAN. Thank you. Thank you, Mr. Chairman.

Chairman TOM DAVIS. Thank you.

Mr. Issa.

Mr. ISSA. Thank you, Mr. Chairman.

I would like to continue right along that same line, but switch for a moment to the nuclear threat. I heard that, for what little information it has given me, I some 30 years ago was in bomb disposal, went through nuclear-biological-chemical training, just enough to understand that everything you are mentioning pretty much was the cold war solution.

So to say that we have something to deal with hundreds of thousands of people that might be affected, even by a rather low technology dirty bomb, is not to say anything terribly new. I saw your head shaking. So I don't think we have to go further into that.

After September 11th, and particularly after October when we began realizing that there would be followon threats, and certainly after July 7th, we are all aware that al Qaeda has not gone out of business, and if they can attack greater London, which is far more fortified than the United States, they will be back here. Why is it we have nothing that can deal with, even a small amount for the first responders, and for the hospital personnel who would also be suffering, why is it we have nothing that is going to dramatically reduce the effects of low-level—let me rephrase that—of radiation sufficient to give radiation sickness or death today? Iodide doesn't get you there.

Mr. SIMONSON. I agree with that. This has been, Congressman, one of my great frustrations since——

Mr. ISSA. We are here to relieve your frustrations.

Mr. SIMONSON. Good. [Laughter.]

Since beginning work in this area, a lot was done in the civil defense movement, in the 1950's, the 1960's, that was disassembled in the 1970's and 1980's. There has not been an enormous amount of work, basic and applied research, on countermeasures against radiation. Funding for the Government's agencies that do that sort of work, like the Armed Forces Radiobiology Research Institute, are pretty much level.

We sought to add to that. We infused funds, Dr. Fauci's institute did, into AFRRI to begin work there to try and develop more of these things. But it takes some time. Like you, I don't think this is a satisfactory state of affairs. We are moving, I think, cautiously but with deliberate speed to remediate it.

Mr. ISSA. OK. Just following up one more on that, yesterday we had a rather lengthy hearing chaired by the chairman here on entrepreneurs and the Government and how to make it more entrepreneurial. We even had the former Speaker of the House sitting in your seat. One of the all agreed on by everybody on the panel was that when you put out a request for entrepreneurial behavior, which to me is risk taking, with the hopes of a return but no guarantee, that the one thing Government has to do is follow through on that promise, meaning, if you say develop radiation or biological vaccines, antidotes, treatments that are effective and reach a standard, we will buy from one of you. Not from all of you. It is a contest. First man to the moon wins, all the others just get leftover capsules sitting in space.

We have already done that, companies have made these investments. One of the next panels, or the entire next panel, is going to be all about people who made those. And now we are sitting here saying—what was it you said, chairman, engaged to be engaged? We are in this position of engaged to be engaged. When will we say, we are going to buy at least enough doses of radiation sickness for the nuclear power plants we expect to be building in the years to come? At least for things which domestically might happen, which we are going to need to be ready for, that we have never been ready for. And then by the way, more doses if we believe that there is a threat and positioning them where they do good.

When is that engagement to be engaged going to become an engagement date?

Mr. SIMONSON. Once the draft request for proposal is published, that will lay out a time line which I think will be responsive to your question. I can't give it to you right now, because it hasn't been published. But once it is, it will be clear in that document.

All I can tell you is, I have certain limitations on me, what I can say about Federal acquisitions, when we are contemplating one. But I can leave you with the assurance that no one is more concerned about this than I am. This is something that we focus on every day at our place. I know it does not always seem satisfactory to the industry.

Mr. ISSA. And at the risk of seeming like Sam Donaldson, a very quick followup. We live in a 2-year world here in Congress. We can only provide you money for 2 years, and after that it is a promise to promise money, and we deal around that.

Can you give us a range outside of your RFP of when effectively, you expect to have delivery of drugs, if they exist, to deal with each of these areas, in the case of radiation, in the case of this draft RFP? Can you just give us a date? Is it greater than this Congress? Is it beyond the next Congress? Will it be after Senator Hillary Clinton leaves office? I just need to know a range. I know that is open to so much questioning.

Mr. SIMONSON. I would say within the life of this Congress, there will be progress, as there has been progress. That is as far as I can go on that.

Mr. ISSA. Yes, Doctor.

Dr. FAUCI. Again, as I mentioned, myself and my agency are responsible for the research that goes into that. But the question you asked, Mr. Issa, of Mr. Simonson really does relate to the success or failure of the research to prove in a pivotal study that this is FDA licensable. That is an issue that is sometimes not fully understood. Because there is more than just having the money. Do you have a product that is going to, in a clinical trial, show to be effective in what you want it to be effective with, so that it would pass the criteria of something that would be FDA licensable to go into the Stockpile.

Now, that is not an excuse for any slowness or fastness. But that is something that really is not understood, that just because there is a product out there doesn't necessarily mean it could be bought to put into the stockpile. There has to be at least the pathway toward what will be FDA approval.

Having said that, if I might just take an extra minute to point something out in response to the question that the chairman asked when I showed that last slide, he asked a very relevant question: is there anything on there for radiation? The reason that there isn't is that we are very far advanced, when you think in terms of microbial and toxin threats. The reason for that is that for decades, we have been preparing for naturally emerging microbes.

So we have the apparatus in place, we have the scientists there, we have the people interested in it. And we do it every day. Infections emerge every day that might be a worse threat than a deliberately released microbe. That is not the case with some other areas of defense countermeasures.

And Mr. Simonson mentioned the issue of the gaps that have been left following the cold war about radiation. We have to almost start from square one. We have to look at what we have, we have to get the indication for licensure, and then we have to go and do the research, research on issues that were never considered when we had nuclear holocaust threats, because there really wasn't much concern about the after-effects of it. It was either you blow up a city or not. It is a totally different picture now, which is the reason why the research is taking time.

So I hope that at least partially answers your question about predicting a timeframe.

Mr. ISSA. It does partially answer it. Thank you, Mr. Chairman.

Chairman TOM DAVIS. Thank you very much.

Mr. Davis.

Mr. DAVIS OF ILLINOIS. Thank you very much, Mr. Chairman.

Dr. Vitko, one of the jobs of the Department of Homeland Security is to identify a material threat to the American people from bioterrorism. You have testified that one of the challenges of the task is that the list of potential threats is quite long. The Department has responded to this challenge by focusing its list on the specific agents deemed to be the most dangerous and credible threats; and of course to me, that makes a lot of sense.

Another way to address the multitude of potential threats is to shore up the basic public health infrastructure and respond to all threats. Core public health functions include communication, surveillance and emergency response. The problem is that the basic public health system is not fully functional. For example, only a handful of States have the capacity to deliver and distribute products from the Strategic National Stockpile. There are also major gaps in laboratory capacity and personnel.

My question is, do you agree that a strong public health system is critical to responding to many of the different agents of bioterrorism?

Dr. VITKO. Absolutely. A strong public health system is the key to any biodefense that we have.

Mr. DAVIS OF ILLINOIS. What would you say that the Department of Homeland Security has done, or what is the Department doing to explain the need for public health investment to the public and of course to the administration?

Dr. VITKO. The Department of Homeland Security's responsibility here, as you know, is an overall coordination and response to terrorist events with the National Response Plan.

Mr. DAVIS OF ILLINOIS. I am sorry, I am having a little difficulty hearing.

Dr. VITKO. I am sorry, Mr. Davis. I was saying that the Department has responsibilities at multiple levels. One is to coordinate the overall response through the National Response Plan. In there, there are specific annexes that deal with, in fact, biological response, in which HHS has a lead under ESF 8 in those activities, emergency support function 8.

We also work very closely with HHS and with the other members of an interagency team in a policy coordinating committee on the Homeland Security Council on Biodefense, in which we look at the integrated aspects of a defense and address key issues, such as mass casualty response, the need and ways to improve that. And we are part of a team of working with them to help identify the key areas to emphasize and develop.

Mr. DAVIS OF ILLINOIS. Does the Department have a position on $130 million in proposed cuts to State and local health departments for bioterrorism preparedness?

Dr. VITKO. I don't know if the Department has an official position. I have not been asked that. I believe we would say that we support HHS fully on what they are doing.

Mr. DAVIS OF ILLINOIS. Does the Department then have an advocacy responsibility to point out that which it understands to be need?

Dr. VITKO. Yes, the Department does have such an advocacy responsibility. And one of the ways that we exercise that is through large scale exercises, barring actual events. As you know, we have just conducted Top Off III as an exercise. In there, the influence of mass casualty response clearly comes up. We work then through the various interagency committees to identify what those needs are, to look for innovative ways to address those and to tackle those and lay out a road map for getting there.

Mr. DAVIS OF ILLINOIS. Would you have any way, would you venture to suggest any assessment of how the American public is responding to threats of bioterrorism?

Dr. VITKO. I have no formal insight in that, in the sense of being able to gauge the full American public. Clearly, it is a concern that is held by many. At the same time, barring an actual event, one tries to balance that in executing their daily lives. It is something they are counting on us as a country to have something there for them, if something bad should happen. But I do not think they are dwelling on it on a daily basis.

Mr. DAVIS OF ILLINOIS. Thank you very much, Mr. Chairman. I have no further questions.

Chairman TOM DAVIS. Thank you very much.

Mr. Shays.

Mr. SHAYS. Thank you, Mr. Chairman, for holding this hearing on a very important subject.

I am going to make a statement to which I then want to respond to questions, Mr. Secretary, that goes to you, basically. During the House debate on the BioShield bill, I expressed concern over the provision that allowed for the use of unapproved vaccines and treatments by military personnel. Testimony before the National Security Subcommittee by the Gulf war veterans confirmed the Department of Defense [DOD], had consistently failed to meet basic requirements to inform recipients about investigational drugs or keep adequate medical records.

Now, the mandatory DOD anthrax program only built on that sorry record, relying on a dated vaccine formulation tested and approved only for protection against cutaneous exposure, not against weaponized or aerosolized anthrax. A Federal court has enjoined the use of the vaccine in a mandatory program due to flaws in the Food and Drug Administration approval process.

And this is my key point, rather than rely on the BioShield to develop a modern anthrax vaccine, the Pentagon chose to rely on another provision of the law permitting the Department of Health and Human Services to grant "emergency use authorization" for continued use of the now "unapproved" anthrax vaccine, albeit in a voluntary program.

So these are my questions. First, did the Department of Health and Human Services have access to the classified November 2004 intelligence community assessment of the anthrax threat?

Mr. SIMONSON. Yes.

Mr. SHAYS. Second, did HHS agree with the Pentagon's conclusion about the nature of the threat our troops faced from anthrax attacks?

Mr. SIMONSON. We did not undertake our own review of their conclusions.

Mr. SHAYS. Did you agree with them?

Mr. SIMONSON. We accepted the Department of Defense's conclusions.

Mr. SHAYS. So you agreed with them?

Mr. SIMONSON. We accepted them.

Mr. SHAYS. Has the authorization for anthrax and the congressional concern changed any HHS policies regarding future requests for emergency use authorization?

Mr. SIMONSON. No.

Mr. SHAYS. So there is no change in policy at all?

Mr. SIMONSON. No, other than that, as I mentioned in the past——

Mr. SHAYS. Why was it necessary? Why did they need to come to you if they had simply made it voluntary? Why did they need to come to you for an emergency program, since you have the authority to do it? They have the authority—do they not have the authority if it is for a voluntary program?

Mr. SIMONSON. It is not clear to me how they would do it as a voluntary program but as an EUA. I suppose they could do it as a treatment IND, but the mechanism for doing that is extremely cumbersome. We wanted to make very sure that the program that we were authorizing allowed members of the Armed Services to decline to take the vaccine. It has been very clear, and as far as I can tell, that part of the program has been very effective.

Mr. SHAYS. Right.

Mr. SIMONSON. Our concern was to make the vaccine available to members who voluntarily wanted to take it. The Department of Defense represented to us that while in the field, it was very common for senior officials, including Dr. Winkenwerter, to hear, when are you going to make this vaccine available to us?

And as I think I mentioned to you before, our view was, Secretary Thompson's view and my view was, if we were in that battlefield, we would want the option to take this vaccine. So we accepted the Department of Defense's determination, but we issued the EUA in a way that was consistent, we think, with the spirit of the request.

Mr. SHAYS. And what kind of requirements, and I would agree that the voluntary nature of it is its saving grace. I do agree that if people want to use it, they should have that capability.

But tell me, what demands and oversight do you have over the Department's explanation to its servicemen and women about the voluntary nature of it?

Mr. SIMONSON. There is an agreed-upon document that states all of the conditions, in very clear language, to the servicemen, to the potential vaccinee. That was approved by the Food and Drug Administration before it could be used by DOD.

Mr. SHAYS. Thank you very much. Thank you, Mr. Chairman.

Chairman TOM DAVIS. Thank you.

Mrs. Maloney.

Mrs. MALONEY. Thank you for having this hearing. I would like to ask Stewart Simonson or Dr. Fauci, the general question on the BioShield progress, the material threat assessment was done in four areas, yet only two RFPs have been issued on the material threat assessments, and why have the other two RFPs not been issued.

But I would like to go back to the questioning also that Ranking Member Waxman had on the BioShield anthrax vaccine purchase program. This is an issue that is very important to me. We have suffered anthrax attacks in the district that I represent in New York. Apparently, you signed an $877 million contract with one company, VaxGen, to procure the 75 million doses of anthrax vaccine, but you do not expect to get that until 2006.

I understand it is a company that has never done this type of research before, and what is this vaccine that is so much better than the stop-gap purchase of 5 million doses of an older, less effective vaccine for $125 million from a second company, I believe it was BioPort? Mr. Waxman mentioned that possibly we should not have used BioShield funding for the stop-gap purchase.

But I find it, I would like to know, why are we going to a company that has never done anthrax or have a track record in producing it? And then you go to another company that can do it at a lesser degree or whatever. Could you explain that contract to me? Why are we going to a company, why did we need the stop-gap, why couldn't the first company—you understand what I'm saying.

Mr. SIMONSON. Yes, sure.

First, VaxGen has done work with this particular type of product. They have an R&D contract with Dr. Fauci's institute, so they are not novices in the field of recombinant protective antigens. The idea is to develop a next generation vaccine. We have been advised by a number of scientific entities, including the Institute of Medicine, that there is a need for a new anthrax vaccine, using 21st century technologies.

So this is what we are doing. We are trying——

Mrs. MALONEY. And VaxGen has produced other anthrax vaccines?

Mr. SIMONSON. No, they have work underway to produce anthrax vaccine. They have a research and development contract with Dr. Fauci's institute.

It is a small biotech firm. But I think you will see, ma'am, that this is going to be the story of Project BioShield. We will be working with the smaller biotech——

Mrs. MALONEY. What other vaccines have they developed in the past?

Mr. SIMONSON. There is no vaccine that they have developed for anthrax that has been licensed. This is a small——

Mrs. MALONEY. Have they developed any vaccines?

Mr. SIMONSON. Not that have been licensed, no.

Mrs. MALONEY. No.

Mr. SIMONSON. But I have to tell you, this will be a fairly commonplace thing with BioShield. The large pharmaceutical and biotech firms are not interested in this work. Dr. Fauci can tell you a little about the market realities of these vaccine and countermeasure production programs. We are going to be working consistently with these smaller firms, and it is going to require an enormous amount of Government effort to get this product licensed.

But there will be good that comes from that. We will build infrastructure and expertise——

Mrs. MALONEY. So no other company wanted to bid on it?

Mr. SIMONSON. There were other bids, yes.

Mrs. MALONEY. And did they have a track record in producing——

Mr. SIMONSON. They were similar types of companies.

Mrs. MALONEY. They had never produced anthrax before, the other companies that bid on it, anthrax vaccine?

Mr. SIMONSON. I am restricted a little in what I can say under the procurement rules, but they were similar types of companies. These were not big pharma companies.

Mrs. MALONEY. I would just be interested in why this company, you believe, can come up with it when they have no track record.

Mr. SIMONSON. This was subject to a very extensive technical review within the Department of Health and Human Services, experts both within and without Government. We work with what we have. We send out RFPs, we get proposals back and we review them and do the best we can with it.

Mrs. MALONEY. OK. I would like to see the proposals and look at them.

Mr. SIMONSON. OK.

Mrs. MALONEY. Also, there was a report that came out about 2 weeks ago from some research group in San Francisco. They were talking about the RFP for botulinum antitoxin, which apparently is very deadly, it could go into the milk supply and hurt many people. What are we doing on that? This report, I don't know if it is correct or not, said we had not done an RFP or reacted to this particular threat.

Mr. SIMONSON. We have a number of botulinum antitoxin programs underway. I assume you are referring to the article that came out of Stanford.

Mrs. MALONEY. Yes, that is the one.

Mr. SIMONSON. We have a program that has just been completed which took plasma that was created during the early 1990's and finished that into botulinum antitoxin, and we have a second botulinum antitoxin program that is underway right now. An RFP, in fact, I think goes out later today or tomorrow.

Mrs. MALONEY. Oh, really, today?

Mr. SIMONSON. Yes, later today or tomorrow.

Mrs. MALONEY. Then my first question on the material threat assessment, I am glad you have done them. But I read that only two RFPs have gone out, when we need to have four going out. I just would like your response to that.

Mr. SIMONSON. Well, I am not sure that is accurate. As I said, I think the botulinum one went out or will be going out in the next couple of days.

There is a period of time that occurs between when the material threat assessment is given and when the RFP is done. The RFPs are very complicated instruments. It is the nature of the document.

Mrs. MALONEY. But actually two have gone out, one is going out today and there is a fourth that needs to go out, right?

Mr. SIMONSON. Right.

Mrs. MALONEY. My time is up. Thank you.

Chairman TOM DAVIS. Thank you very much. Ms. Watson.

Ms. WATSON. I too want to add my thanks, Mr. Chairman, to you for having this hearing.

We have been talking about the chemical and radiological and biological threats and protecting the general public against an attack. We have experienced the anthrax attack when it reared its ugly head in the Hart Building and in the Longworth Building.

So I want to focus on the responsibility that we have to the general public. I think legislators must be held accountable for the organizational structure that we create and the procurement processes that we devise. As we move forward with our BioShield programs, it is imperative that we as lawmakers take all bias and politics out of the funding and jurisdiction. We must also be cautious and informed on the proper levels of preparedness.

In terms of public health, too little is far greater a risk than too much. The difficult job that Congress approaches is making decisions based on well-constructed calculations, not on the emotional or political agendas that can arise when a threat or an implied threat is aimed at our country.

So I too would want to know about this company that we are going after and I have learned from Roche, the pharmaceutical company, that 7 million courses of treatment, and I guess this treatment has to do with Tamiflu, we had a hearing last week on it, are available for sale from next year's production. I see the flu as being a threat to the public's health.

So I really feel, Mr. Chairman, that oversight needs to be periodical and continuous. We need to know and you can comment, let me be sure I am addressing this to the right person, I guess it is the Honorable Stewart Simonson, you can comment as to the level of preparedness that we are positioned at at this particular time.

I want to be sure that as you analyze, as you review these various proposals that you are getting, I just heard it said that not a whole lot of companies responded, so we are going with the one that has. I want to make sure that what they are presenting us with is the best and that it will guarantee that we can have a BioShield stand in the way of attacks that would be made on our general public.

So with that said, I am listening very closely to hear evidence that we are prepared, or we are getting there. Thank you very much, and thank you very much, Mr. Chairman.

Chairman TOM DAVIS. Thank you very much.

Any other questions? Mr. Van Hollen.

Mr. VAN HOLLEN. Mr. Chairman, I just want to first apologize to the witnesses for being late. I am on two other committees that have markups this morning, Judiciary and Education and Workforce. I look forward to reading your testimony and listening to the next panel as much as I can.

Thank you, Mr. Chairman, for the hearing.

Chairman TOM DAVIS. Thank you.

Ms. Norton, any questions?

Ms. NORTON. None, thank you, Mr. Chairman.

Chairman TOM DAVIS. OK, thank you all for bearing with us. We will dismiss this panel at this point, take a 2-minute recess as we convene the next panel. That panel will have Mr. Robert Kramer, the CEO of BioPort Corp.; Mr. Richard Hollis, the CEO of Hollis-Eden Pharmaceuticals; and Mr. Gerald Epstein, the senior fellow for science and security, Homeland Security Program, Center for Strategic and International Studies.

[Recess.]

Chairman TOM DAVIS. We are going to our second panel. Again, we have Mr. Robert Kramer, the CEO of BioPort Corp.; Richard Hollis, the CEO of Hollis-Eden Pharmaceuticals; and Dr. Gerald Epstein, the senior fellow for science and security, Homeland Security Programs, Center for Strategic and International Studies.

I know Mr. Issa wanted to be here to introduce you, Mr. Hollis, but I am going to go ahead and swear you in. I am going to have to run upstairs for a couple of minutes in between and will have one of the other Members take the chair. Please rise and raise your right hands.

[Witnesses sworn.]

Chairman TOM DAVIS. Thank you very much.

Dr. Kramer, we will start with you and then we will go to Mr. Hollis and then to Dr. Epstein. Thanks for being with us and thanks for your patience.

STATEMENTS OF ROBERT G. KRAMER, PRESIDENT AND CHIEF EXECUTIVE OFFICER, BIOPORT CORP.; RICHARD B. HOLLIS, CHAIRMAN AND CHIEF EXECUTIVE OFFICER, HOLLIS-EDEN PHARMACEUTICALS; AND GERALD L. EPSTEIN, SENIOR FELLOW FOR SCIENCE AND SECURITY, HOMELAND SECURITY PROGRAM, CENTER FOR STRATEGIC AND INTERNATIONAL STUDIES

STATEMENT OF ROBERT G. KRAMER

Mr. KRAMER. Chairman Davis, thank you, as well as the other members of the committee, for the opportunity to share some comments with you this afternoon. You have a copy of my written testimony and I am not going to read it, but rather just make a few general comments and summary observations.

These comments are going to be focused on the recent decisions by the Government related to the procurement of vaccines to protect Americans from the threat of anthrax and botulinum. But I believe they have application to all other threats that are being considered. BioPort Corp. manufactures BioThrax, the only FDA-licensed product for the prevention of anthrax. Our company has a more than 70 year history of development, testing, licensure and commercialization of biologic products.

Since privatizing the company in 1998, we have upheld our long-term commitment to the Federal Government to be a reliable partner for anthrax vaccine as a critically needed biodefense countermeasure. Since 1998, BioThrax has been used to protect over 1.3 million military members serving our country throughout the world. To be clear, this means over 5 million doses of BioThrax have been administered to these military personnel.

The product itself has been licensed since 1970. It has been the subject of numerous safety and efficacy studies, as has been well documented, one of the most thoroughly reviewed vaccines. The most recent review was done by the National Academy of Sciences Institute of Medicine panel, which published this finding in March 2002, which sought to answer two questions: is the vaccine safe and is it effective? Very clearly, the answer to both those questions was yes.

As a company, we have submitted more than four proposals since 2001, detailing our commitment, our capability and willingness to provide an unlimited number of licensed anthrax vaccine doses to the Strategic National Stockpile. Rather than take us up on any of those proposals, the Department of Health and Human Services has recently awarded a nearly $1 billion contract for an experimental vaccine that has been used in fewer than 1,000 recipients. I will repeat: our vaccine has been used in over 1.3 million patients. The experimental product they have invested over $1 billion in has been used in less than 1,000.

This policy decision by HHS raises serious concerns about the Government's commitment to the underlying goals of Project BioShield. Let me be real specific in that regard. One of the important goals of BioShield is to increase the number of biodefense companies in the United States. By prohibiting proven companies with proven products from participating in contracts like the 75 million dose contract for anthrax vaccine, the Government will eliminate biodefense companies, not increase them, and will not encourage them to participate in taking the risks that we have all talked about this morning and this afternoon necessary to bring products to the market.

A related goal of BioShield was to create a strong manufacturing base to further avoid a similar crisis to what occurred in October 2004 with regard to the flu vaccine supply. The Government excluded from the outset and by design the only licensed anthrax vaccine from participating or competing for the 75 million dose order.

Unfortunately, this experience is not only occurring with respect to anthrax vaccine, but also for vaccines to protect against botulinum. The U.S. Government, in announcing its intention to purchase an early stage experimental botulinum vaccine from a sole source eliminated several competing manufacturers and technologies and reduced the potential for ultimately acquiring a safe and effective vaccine targeted at this threat.

A third Project BioShield goal was to increase the uses for licensed products. Yet with respect to anthrax vaccine, the purchase of an experimental product does nothing to accomplish this.

The last goal that I will mention has to do with the Government's commitment to buy best in class medical countermeasures at competitive prices. Again, HHS intends to procure a vaccine for nearly all of the future stockpile needs for anthrax from a single supplier at a cost higher than it was proposed for the existing FDA-licensed anthrax vaccine.

Further, phase 1 studies provide no evidence that the experimental product provides any improvement in terms of safety or efficacy over the currently licensed product, BioThrax. In fact, the published data illustrate that it took an additional dose plus an additional 30 days for the experimental product to provide a comparable protection to that with BioThrax.

Despite these results, HHS distributed a news release in March 2004 touting the experimental vaccine as being proven to be safer and more effective than BioThrax. HHS subsequently withdrew this news release from its Web site when they were under inquiry from Senator Grassley.

I will add that had a company such as ours or anyone on this panel made such remarks, you can be assured that the FDA would have demanded an immediate retraction and withdrawal and correction of such statements.

HHS has staked the Nation's protection against the No. 1 biologic threat on an experimental product. It is clear to me and many of my colleagues in this industry the shortcomings that I have discussed and articulated. One way to help prevent these shortcomings from reoccurring is to provide some early oversight into the BioShield procurement process. The evaluation and eventual procurement of products such as anthrax vaccine is extremely complex and requires expertise from an open, independent, multi-disciplinary review. The risks of failure for products such as these are too great and the costs of these failures are simply too large to continue to do otherwise.

When you add to that the importance of these products, namely, they protect and save lives, in my opinion there is no Government procurement challenge greater than what is at stake today with Project BioShield. It therefore requires a sound, discipline approach that includes expert representation from medical, scientific, regulatory and compliance personnel to assist with these key decisions.

In closing, it is essential to recognize that our industry is very young, very fragile and very much dependent upon a unique customer, the U.S. Government, for a strong partnership to bring these kinds of products to market. Unless we do so, the industry will be characterized by companies that have a lack of proven record, they will be in it for the short run and they will not be a viable long-term partner for the U.S. Government.

Thank you again for allowing me to share with you my comments and I look forward to answering any questions you have.

[The prepared statement of Mr. Kramer follows:]

ROBERT G. KRAMER
PRESIDENT AND CHIEF EXECUTIVE OFFICER
BIOPORT CORPORATION

BEFORE THE UNITED STATE HOUSE OF REPRESENTATIVES
COMMITTEE ON GOVERNMENT REFORM

REGARDING THE
IMPLEMENTATION OF PROJECT BIOSHIELD
AND THE STATE OF BIODEFENSE
IN THE UNITED STATES

JULY 14, 2005

Chairman Davis, Congressman Waxman and Members of the Committee, it is an honor for me to testify before you today regarding the current state of the implementation of the Project BioShield Act of 2004. I am Bob Kramer, President and Chief Executive Officer of BioPort Corporation. Let me begin by thanking the Committee for its leadership in this critical public health and national security area. The bipartisan work of this Committee's members, including the leadership of Chairman Davis and Congressman Waxman, in the passage of the Project BioShield Act of 2004 was a credit to each of you. I applaud President Bush for his vision in announcing Project BioShield in his 2003 State of the Union Address. I come before you today to testify on issues of concern to industry regarding the implementation of BioShield. I will reflect on these challenges using anthrax and botulinum vaccines as examples, but I believe they are lessons that can be applied to multiple threats.

BioPort Corporation manufactures BioThrax, the only FDA licensed vaccine for the prevention of anthrax. Our company's history is a successful story of the privatization of the State of Michigan's vaccine production laboratory, which had a 70-year history rich in the development, manufacture and licensure of biologic products. Since privatizing this company in 1998, we have upheld our long-term commitment to the federal government to be a reliable partner for anthrax vaccine as a critically needed biodefense countermeasure. Since 1998, BioThrax has been used to protect more than 1.3 million U.S. military members serving our country around the world. To be clear, this means that over five million doses of BioThrax have been administered in the past seven years. BioThrax and BioPort are proven. Both the product and the company have performed well over time. A safety profile established in more than a million recipients should not be ignored. Yet the largest contract let under Project BioShield has been awarded for the procurement of an experimental anthrax vaccine administered to fewer than 1,000 recipients. At the same time, the federal government has signed a contract for only five million doses of the FDA licensed anthrax vaccine, and despite all attempts, appears to have only a luke-warm interest in adding meaningful quantities of this vaccine to the Strategic National Stockpile.

It is with this reality that BioPort Corporation must weigh the costs of continuing to manufacture this FDA approved product. As we all know, the principal customer for biodefense countermeasures are government agencies such as the departments of Homeland Security, Health and Human Services and Defense. For a company such as ours, it is critical that the government provides a firm commitment for these products to justify the continued resources necessary to maintain consistent and compliant production facilities and operations. Over the past four years, BioPort has demonstrated its commitment to produce BioThrax at large scale and at favorable pricing. In that effort, we have submitted no fewer than four proposals to decision makers at the Department of Health and Human Services regarding our ability to meet our nation's requirements for anthrax vaccine. As early as December of 2001, BioPort presented HHS with a proposal that could have provided a hundred million doses of licensed anthrax vaccine for the SNS by this time. The notion of "build it and they will come" does not apply to vaccine manufacturing in the biodefense field. The costs are too high, and the risks are too great for the companies and products, particularly when sales are highly dependent upon the U.S. Government procurement decisions.

As you are aware, Project BioShield has several implicit goals. The first goal is to increase the number of biodefense companies in the United States. And yet, with respect to anthrax vaccine, there remains only one FDA licensed supplier, BioPort, and only one experimental, non-FDA licensed vaccine. According to public statements made by HHS representatives, the experimental vaccine, under the best case scenario, will not be delivered to the stockpile until fiscal 2007, and even then, will likely not be licensed before 2009, if ever. And most importantly, while described as a "next generation" vaccine, the experimental anthrax vaccine will not have any clear advantages over the existing, FDA licensed vaccine in terms of safety, efficacy, administration or production.

The second implicit goal of BioShield is to create a strong, diversified manufacturing base to avoid another crisis similar to that which occurred in October 2004 with the flu vaccine supply. Again, the procurement process for the anthrax vaccine was designed to limit rather than expand the manufacturing base. The government excluded, from the outset and by design, the only licensed anthrax vaccine manufacturer. Moreover, in the procurement process, the government down selected several other competing manufacturers, resulting in a procurement of a single experimental anthrax vaccine produced at a single plant. By this process, the government has created an environment designed to eliminate a proven product and a proven manufacturer. Thus, the government has truly ignored the bird-in-the-hand while turning to the one-in-the-bush, thereby potentially REDUCING the number of suppliers and amount of countermeasure production capacity. This is precisely the opposite outcome from what was intended under BioShield.

Unfortunately, this experience is being replayed in another government agency's sole source solicitation of an experimental vaccine for the prevention of botulinum, another Category A threat. The U.S. Government, in announcing its intention to purchase an early stage experimental botulinum vaccine from a single-source, eliminated several competing manufacturers and technologies and reduced the potential for ultimately acquiring a safe and effective vaccine targeted at this threat. Again, BioPort as well as others, has been excluded from this procurement. In our view, this is extraordinary given that BioPort is the only manufacturer that has produced an IND botulinum vaccine for government use over the past 20 years and has notified the government that it stands ready to develop several potential botulinum vaccines with timelines well within those required. Yet the government set specifications in its solicitation expressly designed to eliminate all potential manufacturers -- save one. We fail to understand the government's implementation philosophy given the underlying objective of Project BioShield and the importance of marshalling our nation's resources to develop these critical countermeasures.

Third, Project BioShield is designed to increase the uses for licensed products. Yet, with respect to anthrax vaccine, the purchase of the experimental product does not expand protection to either children or the elderly. Moreover, while the government has stated that a true, "next generation" anthrax vaccine that meets the government's requirements would have a simpler mechanism of delivery (e.g., a skin patch), have a longer shelf-life, not require cold storage, and would provide immunity against a number of lethal toxins caused by the anthrax bacteria, the experimental vaccine has none of these characteristics. This begs the question why the government has committed to an investment of more than $1 billion in a vaccine that does not achieve its own criteria.

Finally, the government, through BioShield, intends to encourage deployment of the "best in class" countermeasures at competitive prices. And yet again, it took the government until May 5, 2005 - over three and a half years from the anthrax attacks in 2001 - to create a stockpile of FDA licensed anthrax vaccine of 5 million doses, despite the clear requirement to stockpile enough vaccine for 25 million Americans. BioPort has prepared and submitted four proposals to HHS over the last four years to supply FDA licensed vaccine to the stockpile at a cost LOWER than the experimental vaccine (and without the $1 billion federal investment). Yet, HHS intends to procure experimental vaccine for nearly all of the future stockpile from a single supplier at a cost higher than that proposed for the existing FDA licensed anthrax vaccine. Further, the Phase I studies provides no evidence that the experimental vaccine provides any improvement in terms of safety or efficacy over BioThrax. In fact, the published data illustrate that it took both an additional dose and an additional month for the experimental product to provide comparable protection to that of BioThrax. The data also demonstrated a higher rate of systemic reactions than those found with BioThrax. Despite these results, HHS distributed a news release in March 2004 touting the experimental product as safer and more effective. Upon inquiry from Senator Grassley, HHS withdrew the news release from its website in tacit recognition that the news release was inaccurate.

Thus, in each of the implicit goals of Project BioShield, at least with respect to anthrax and botulinum vaccines, Project BioShield has come up short. Considering that fully one-third of the $3.4 billion dollars in currently available funding from Project BioShield has been dedicated to anthrax vaccine, this result is clearly troubling. Despite the availability of an FDA licensed competing vaccine technology, HHS has staked the nation's protection against the number one biologic threat on an experimental product that may never be licensed by the FDA. This has made the government and the nation's security against anthrax attacks highly dependent on an unproven technology. Moreover, the government awarded the primary anthrax vaccine stockpile contract to a single vendor, thereby making the nation's security against such attacks dependent on only one manufacturer.

Having highlighted a number of issues, I would like to make a recommendation intended to improve the procurement process involving Project Bioshield funds. The evaluation and eventual procurement of products such as anthrax vaccine is extremely complex and requires the expertise of a multi-disciplined review. Biopharmaceutical companies are managed and operated by multiple disciplines. We count on experienced professionals from the fields of science, medicine, operations, regulatory and compliance to participate in key decisions related to product development. The procurement process for vaccines and other medical countermeasures should follow suit. There is a fundamental need for early oversight in the BioShield procurement process. The risks of failure are too great and the cost of failure is too large to simply continue to operate in a vacuum. Ours is an exacting and demanding business with enormous risk associated. When you add to that the importance of the product candidates involved and the potential to protect and save lives, I cannot imagine a government procurement challenge that is greater than what is at stake with Project BioShield. It therefore requires a sound, disciplined approach that includes expert representation from the medical, scientific, regulatory, and threat assessment perspectives, and is conducted in a manner open to the public. Each procurement should be focused on assuring multiple technologies, multiple companies and multi-year commitments to industry partners. Implementation of a transparent, multi-disciplinary approach to procurements would also go a long way in allowing the government to build credibility with industry.

In closing, it is essential to recognize that our industry is young and dependent, to a great extent, on a unique customer—the U.S. Government. In the absence of a strong and consistent commitment from that customer, the industry will be characterized by companies that lack a proven track record and that have an inability to sustain over a long period of time. I would restate that BioPort Corporation finds itself at a critical juncture in terms of its ability and willingness to commit resources to a product that lacks a committed customer. I respectfully submit my comments and am willing to answer any questions that members may have.

Mr. SHAYS [presiding]. Thank you, Mr. Kramer.
Mr. Hollis.

STATEMENT OF RICHARD B. HOLLIS

Mr. HOLLIS. Mr. Vice Chairman, members of the committee, my name is Richard Hollis. I am chairman and CEO of Hollis-Eden Pharmaceuticals, the manufacturer of NEUMUNE, the first medical countermeasure being developed to address acute radiation syndrome or radiation sickness as a result of nuclear terrorism and exposure to radiation. I ask that my entire statement be entered into the record.

This morning, the chairman opened up the meeting with some chilling videos about the nuclear threat and also in yesterday's press release from Michael Chertoff describing the reorganization of the Department of Homeland Security, he stated: "Of all the catastrophic threats we face, a nuclear attack on our soil would be uniquely threatening to our society." All of the Nation's leaders from the President on down have concluded that the greatest threat to our Nation is nuclear proliferation and nuclear material in the hands of a terrorist.

Recently, during a televised interview, the chairman and vice chairman of the 9/11 Commission both stated that not only is nuclear detonation in one or more of our major cities possible, but it is probable. The death toll from the detonation of a relatively small nuclear device in one or more of our major cities would be devastating.

Medical reports indicate the vast majority of those who are killed, hundreds of thousands would die from acute radiation syndrome. The sad thing about this is the overwhelming majority of these people could be saved if our Government was better prepared to respond to a nuclear scenario.

Now, imagine if you could rapidly distribute a drug to people to give themselves an injection, much like the soldiers do following a chemical attack, and most importantly, imagine up to 90 percent of the people who receive this treatment could survive exposure to radiation. We have a drug in development with the potential to treat acute radiation syndrome that could be in the Strategic National Stockpile as early as next year.

In primate tests done under the Department of Defense oversight using lethal doses of radiation, NEUMUNE has been shown to increase survival rates up to 90 percent. To date, it has no significant side effects. It is inexpensive to manufacture. It can be self-administered in the field without hospitalization. We have opened up an IND with the FDA to initiate our human clinical studies, and we anticipate NEUMUNE could potentially be commercialized with an NDA toward the end of 2006.

There is currently no drug in the stockpile to deal with the acute effects of a nuclear detonation or acute radiation syndrome. Despite this phenomenal progress with NEUMUNE, and the suitability for BioShield contract, we have heard very little from the Federal Government in regard to the procurement of this drug. Without having this commitment, we do not know how to scale our batch sizes, what drug delivery configuration is preferred or how many manufacturers we should validate. All of these activities cost tens of millions of dollars and we have reached the point where decision have to be made or the project risks meaningful delays.

Over 10 months ago, HHS issued a request for information for therapeutics to treat acute radiation syndrome. We were informed that a draft RFP would be issued by July 2005, and to date, we have still heard nothing. More to the point, we don't even understand why the agency is even going through a draft RFP, given the results of the prior RFP process that has already taken over 10 months. During this 10 months, we have incurred tens of millions of dollars in development. It is just more delays and mixed market signals to our investors.

To the best of our knowledge, we are the only company that is close to delivering a drug that meets the requirements for this specific request for proposal. For this reason, earlier this week, Hollis-Eden submitted an unsolicited proposal to allow HHS to immediately procure NEUMUNE for the Strategic National Stockpile. This proposal meets each and every legal requirement for the acceptance under existing law and regulation.

In an environment where BioShield was supposed to stimulate capital investment in companies like ours, delays by HHS have caused Hollis-Eden to lose approximately $600 million in market capitalization. This is just the opposite effect of the intention of what BioShield was supposed to do.

In summary, BioShield, to work effectively, HHS and DHS must define the markets by issuing the threats and what countermeasures are needed to address those threats and how many doses of the drug will be procured. They need to put out RFIs and RFPs for what countermeasures are needed and they need to have an independent scientific review board assess the respondents to the RFIs as to whether the science is feasible and whether the company can deliver in a reasonable period of time and award advance purchase contracts early.

So I would submit to this committee, this is a very important question for me to ask the committee and members, given that the nuclear threat is the greatest threat we face, given that more than a million lives per detonation may be on the line, given that a promising, effective medical countermeasure to acute radiation syndrome is close to fruition and it is now 4 years after September 11th, why is this drug not a top priority to be deployed to protect the American public?

Finally, how will you, our country's leaders, try to explain why so many people unnecessarily, from a nuclear September 11th, when experts are predicting this nightmarish scenario, and we fail to prepare our Nation by providing and forward deploying a drug that could save millions of lives?

Mr. Chairman and Mr. Vice Chairman, it is an honor to be here today. Thank you for the opportunity to be of service to our Nation and homeland security and to protect and safeguard the citizens of our free country. Thank you very much.

[The prepared statement of Mr. Hollis follows:]

'TESTIMONY OF RICHARD B. HOLLIS CHAIRMAN AND CHIEF EXECUTIVE OFFICER, HOLLIS-EDEN PHARMACEUTICALS

BEFORE THE COMMITTEE ON GOVERNMENT REFORM UNITED STATES HOUSE OF REPRESENTATIVES

Oversight Hearing Concerning the Implementation of Project Bioshield

July 14, 2005

Mr. Chairman, Congressman Waxman, distinguished members of the Committee:

Thank you for the opportunity to testify before you today. Before I begin, allow me to thank you personally for your longstanding leadership, both as a Committee and individually, to help safeguard this nation against terrorism, and specifically against the threat posed by weapons of mass destruction. Your Committee has been at the forefront of working to ensure that our federal homeland security programs and policies have been as effective and efficient as possible, including in the area of countering nuclear, biological and chemical terrorist threats.

My name is Richard Hollis. I am Chairman and Chief Executive Officer of Hollis-Eden Pharmaceuticals. Hollis-Eden is a San Diego-based biotechnology company, publicly traded on the NASDAQ stock exchange. Hollis-Eden has under development a number of proprietary immune-regulating hormones, compounds that are key components of the human immune system. We believe that by properly utilizing these hormones, we can help the body to mount an appropriate immune or metabolic response to a host of different diseases or immune system challenges. Specifically, we have developed and tested our compounds for the potential treatment of Acute Radiation Syndrome (ARS), HIV/AIDS, tuberculosis, malaria, cystic fibrosis, rheumatoid arthritis, and multiple sclerosis, among other possible applications.

THE NUCLEAR THREAT

Mr. Chairman, virtually every day brings news of the growing threat posed by nuclear proliferation and by the ongoing efforts of Al Qaeda and other terrorist groups to obtain nuclear weapons. We have seen with the attacks last week in London that the enemy will continue to strike us. Thankfully, they used conventional explosives. But the next time, they might not. We simply cannot afford to take that risk—we must be prepared.

In light of this threat, national security experts routinely cite the threat of nuclear attack by a rogue state like North Korea or Iran or by a terrorist group as the number one security threat facing this country. During the 2004 Presidential Debates, both President Bush and Senator Kerry agreed that the single greatest threat to our nation was a nuclear weapon in the hands of a terrorist. A few weeks ago Governor Tom Kean and your former colleague Lee Hamilton, the leaders of the 9-11 Commission, appeared on "Meet the Press" along with former Senators Sam Nunn, Fred Thompson, and Senate Foreign Relations Chairman Richard Lugar to discuss the threat of nuclear terrorism. At the end of the program, host Tim Russert asked each guest, given all they know about subject of nuclear terrorism, in their best judgment did they think that within their lifetimes they would witness a nuclear bomb going off in an American city? Unfortunately each guest replied in the affirmative.

Governor Kean then elaborated: "Not only do I believe America will experience a nuclear bomb in my lifetime but everyone I have spoken to that is an expert on the subject believes so too." The program also quoted CIA Director Porter Goss when he stated, "It is "only a matter of time before al Qaeda tries to use a chemical, biological or nuclear weapon against the United States."

Most recently, the head of the Domestic Nuclear Detection Office at the Department of Homeland Security, Vayl Oxford, stated that, "A lot of people want to quibble about the nature of the nuclear threat. I tell my people, assume there is a 100 percent chance someone will try to attack us with a nuclear weapon in the next five to 10 years." Similar conclusions have been reached by a number of recent prominent analyses of the threat of a nuclear or radiological attack, including those by Harvard professor Graham Alison, the Monterrey Institute, and the Nuclear Threat Initiative, headed by former Senator Sam Nunn.

These fears are well founded:

- In May 1998, Osama bin Laden issued a statement entitled "The Nuclear Bomb of Islam," proclaiming that Muslims have a duty to acquire nuclear weapons and terrorize the enemies of God, in particular the United States. In an interview with Rahimullah Yousafsai from *ABC News* he stated, "acquiring [nuclear] weapons for the defense of Muslims is a religious duty."
- During the trial of Osama bin Laden for the 1998 US Embassy bombings, prosecution witness Jamal Ahmad al-Fadl detailed his efforts to assist Bin Laden in an attempt to acquire uranium, presumably for the development of nuclear weapons from a source in Khartoum, Sudan, in late 1993 or early 1994.
- The Arabic newspaper *Al-Hayat* reported in late 1998 that bin Laden had made a $30 million deal in Chechnya to purchase twenty nuclear warheads stolen in Russia by Chechen rebels. Bin Laden reportedly gave the contacts in Chechnya $30 million in cash and two tons of opium in exchange for approximately 20 nuclear warheads. Sources stated that bin Laden planned to have the warheads dismantled by his own team of scientists, who would then transform the weapons into "instant nukes" or "suitcase nukes."
- In September 1998, bin Laden's aide, Mamdough Mahmud Salim, was arrested in Munich, Germany on charges of attempting to obtain highly enriched uranium (HEU) in the mid-1990s.
- Director George Tenet told Congress in January 2002 that the United States uncovered rudimentary diagrams of nuclear weapons in a suspected al Qaeda

house in Kabul. According to a CIA report released publicly on January 30, 2002, these "diagrams, while crude, describe the essential components, uranium and high explosives, common to nuclear weapons."

- In November 2001, CNN reported that an Arabic document titled "Superbomb" was found in the home of Abu Khabbab, the codename of a senior al Qaeda official. The document discussed various types of nuclear weapons, the physics of nuclear explosions, the materials needed to make them, and their effects on urban centers.
- Two Pakistani nuclear scientists, Sultan Bashiruddin Mahmood and Chaudiri Abdul Majeed, admitted that they had had long discussions with al Qaeda operatives in August 2001 about the development of nuclear weapons. Pakistani officials told *The Washington Post* that the scientists reportedly admitted meeting with bin Laden, Egyptian Ayman Zawahiri, and two other al Qaeda officials to discuss the procurement of nuclear weapons materials and technology.

LACK OF PREPARATION TO ADDRESS THE NUCLEAR THREAT

The results of a nuclear attack on this nation would be devastating. The Department of Homeland Security's nuclear National Planning Scenario (NNPS) estimates that the number of dead from a terrorist attack on a major U.S. city would be in the hundreds of thousands, possibly reaching one million. Potentially millions more people would become seriously ill.

The reality is that, as of today, the vast majority of these deaths are preventable—assuming we act to prepare the nation to respond to such an attack.

Contrary to popular belief, the majority of the victims of a nuclear attack would die not from the blast but from Acute Radiation Syndrome (ARS). ARS is the result of radiation-induced bone marrow damage. Specifically, ARS is characterized by the loss of infection fighting cells and clotting elements that are produced in bone marrow. This loss of the body's ability to fight infection and prevent bleeding is believed to be the leading cause of sickness and death in the event of a nuclear attack. In fact, some estimates of the medical consequences from a nuclear bomb indicate that ARS would likely kill three to five times as many people as the initial blast.

The British Medical Journal recently estimated that a 12.5 kiloton bomb detonated in New York City would kill at least 50,000 people instantly. But another 200,000 would be expected to die later from ARS and an estimated 700,000 more would become sick from the affects of ARS. The report also states that in a disaster of this magnitude, hospitals and other health care providers would be immediately overwhelmed, leaving the vast majority of victims with few or no treatment options.

There are simply not enough hospital beds to address such a surge. This situation would be compounded by the fact that perhaps millions of "worried well," those who only believe they may have been exposed to radiation, would seek treatment at the same time as those who really do need treatment.

To date, our nation has no workable plan to address the needs of these potentially millions of sick and worried well in the aftermath of a nuclear attack. The key to such a plan is the ability to treat ARS.

If you can manage ARS you can send in first responders. If you cannot, victims will be on their own. If you can manage ARS you can evacuate people in an orderly fashion while radiation levels are subsiding. If you cannot, mass evacuation becomes virtually impossible. If you can treat ARS you can save victims' lives. If you cannot, the nation will have little to offer to victims. In short, if you can effectively treat ARS after a nuclear attack you can save hundreds of thousands of American lives.

Sixty years after the atomic blasts at Nagasaki and Hiroshima, there remains no drug licensed or deployed to treat ARS. The only drugs now available for radiation injury are Potassium Iodide, which helps to prevent thyroid cancer years from the time of exposure, and "chelating" agents like Prussian Blue, which may help rid the body of certain types of radioactive isotopes from fallout, but which do nothing to address initial bone marrow injury, the main cause of ARS.

Senator Robert Byrd (D-WV) specifically asked HHS, in connection with a recent Senate hearing on Project Bioshield, about the status of developing and acquiring effective medical countermeasures to ARS. In response, Assistant Secretary Stewart Simonson stated that HHS had acquired potassium iodide and had the ability to use other, extremely expensive drugs, presently used to treat cancer patients, under an emergency use IND for an off-label indication.

This response ignores the fact that potassium iodide is not a treatment of ARS, but again only helps mitigate the long-term risk of thyroid cancer. Moreover, this response ignores entirely that the cancer treatments referred to in Mr. Simonson's response are not only expensive and have to be refrigerated but also they must be administered by a doctor under highly controlled circumstances with adjunctive therapies such as antibiotics and platelets in a hospital. As stated above, there is no scenario where any one city would have adequate hospital beds to address the surge capacity following detonation of a nuclear device on U.S. soil.

Thankfully, there is an alternative.

THE ANSWER: NEUMUNE, THE WORLD'S FIRST NUCLEAR MEDICALCOUNTERMEASURE

Mr. Chairman, the good news I am here today to deliver to you and the American people is that such a drug is not only possible, but it is at hand. My company, Hollis-Eden is actually on the verge of delivering what we believe will be a monumental medical and historical breakthrough: a drug that can dramatically improve Americans chances for survival in the event of a nuclear attack.

Two weeks after the devastating September 11, 2001 attacks on our country, officials from the Armed Forces Radiobiology Research Institute ("AFRRI"), a research division of the Department of Defense, approached Hollis-Eden and informed us that they wanted to fast track the development of one of our experimental drugs for the treatment of ARS. In some early studies with mice, AFRRI found that our compound coded HE2100 or Neumeune saved literally 100 percent of the lab animals that would have otherwise died from acute radiation exposure. Since that time, AFRRI has continued testing and publishing results in the medical literature on this compound for use in mitigating the effects of ARS.

To date, results of test in over 200 non-human primates treated with NEUMUNE demonstrated the drug to be safe and effective in the treatment of ARS. In one recent trial, 90 percent of the treated primates survived otherwise lethal doses of radiation, while only 55 percent of the untreated group survived. Extrapolating these results using the numbers of people who will be exposed to ARS in a nuclear attack on a major American city shows the dramatic effect this drug could have in reducing the number of casualties in such an event.

Testing to date has shown that the drug is stable at room temperature and can be easily stockpiled. It can be self-administered in the field by victims of such an attack without the need for clinical support, thereby freeing-up medical resources that would otherwise be stretched beyond the breaking point. Moreover, the drug has exhibited no significant side effects. And assuming a contract of sufficient size to offer economies of scale, we believe can provide the drug at a cost akin to that of a standard antibiotic—approximately $75 to $100 per dose regimen.

IMPLEMENTATION OF BIOSHIELD HAS FAILED TO ADEQUATELY ADDRESS THIS THREAT

After a three-and-a-half-year long relationship with the federal government to get such a drug procured and into our civilian and military drug procurement, we have begun to see initial signs that the government is prepared to move forward with procurement of a treatment for ARS.

On May 20 of this year, the Department of Health and Human Services issued a Special Notice, advising of its intent to issue a draft Request for Proposals by the end of this month to acquire a drug for the prevention and/or treatment of Acute Radiation Syndrome. This follows the Department's issuance of a Request for Information notice on October 19th, 2004, which we were happy to respond to. While this is certainly positive, it appears that HHS intends to pursue an extremely conservative approach to procure an ARS therapy and is not utilizing the expedited authorities Congress provided under Project Bioshield.

That said, HHS is well aware based upon the results of the RFI response and market surveys, that there is simply is no other single product that can match the lifesaving abilities of Hollis-Eden's NEUMUNE for the treatment of ARS. Thus, HHS should make use of the authorities under Project Bioshield, or even the typical-FAR authorities, to award a contract to Hollis-Eden as quickly as possible. While there are other products that purport to treat ARS, they are in very early stage of development, only beginning the regulatory process for licensure. Moreover, they are being produced by more or less "virtual" companies that have spent less than $300,000 in the development of their purported treatments based upon public filings. Thus, the very idea that HHS will conduct a competition for a product it knows has no comparable equivalent simply does not make sense.

For this reason, earlier this week, Hollis-Eden has prepared and submitted an unsolicited proposal under Part 15.7 of the Federal Acquisition Regulations to allow HHS to immediately procure NEUMUNE for the SNS. This proposal meets each and every legal requirement for acceptance under existing law and regulation. By promptly evaluating this proposal, and awarding a contract to Hollis-Eden for procurement of adequate supplies of NEUMNE under existing authorities, HHS can assure the nation it is prepared for the scenario that leaders such as Governor Kean and Congressman Hamilton have said is all but inevitable.

We heartily welcome HHS' recent movements to finally address ARS, and look forward to continuing to partner with the federal government to provide the country with safe and effective medical countermeasures to radiation exposure by the prompt review and positive response to our Unsolicited Proposal.

THE FUTURE OF THE BIOSHIELD PROGRAM

With the background of my companys' experience with ARS, I would like to offer a few observations about the implementation of Bioshield and the future of the emerging biological, chemical, and nuclear defense industry.

Many in both the pharmaceutical and national security circles look to Hollis-Eden as a model for the BioShield Program:

- We are, we believe, the first truly new, post 9-11 medical countermeasure to a WMD threat.
- As Bioshield envisions, we have developed this drug almost exclusively with private investment capital and not taxpayer dollars. We have spent and continue to spend tens of millions of dollars to fund expensive trials and other development costs conducted by AFRRI and elsewhere. In fact, we have spent over $100 million to develop NEUMUNE, and we are on the verge of spending millions more for the required pivotal efficacy and safety trials for the drug to qualify for approval, which we believe could be during the first half of 2006.

We have done all of this with no guaranteed market for the product, government or otherwise. Rather, we have developed this drug under the belief and understanding that the federal government would enter into an advanced purchase contract to procure a safe, practical and cost effective drug with the potential to save hundreds of thousands of American lives if a nuclear terrorist incident were to occur in one or more of our cities.

We believe that when Congress passed Project Bioshield it did so with the intent of stimulating the private sector biotechnology and pharmaceutical industries to develop the next-generation of medical countermeasures to WMD.

The bill as described by Dr. Mark McClellan at the 2003 BIO CEO conference was very straightforward and initially very attractive to companies and investors. He described the process as one in which the secretaries of HHS and DHS would collaborate and agree on the major chemical, biological, radiological and nuclear (CBRN) threats and unmet medical needs to those threats. Once the threats were established, HHS would then assess what type of medical countermeasures were needed to address that threat. During the scientific assessment of new technology if the scientific experts thought it was feasible to develop such a countermeasure within <u>eight years</u>, the federal government would enter into an advanced purchase contract with that company committing the federal government to buy the product upon successful FDA approval. Dr. McClellan went on to emphasize that Bioshield advance purchase contracts must be of a size and scope—"hundreds of millions of dollars"—that would be sufficient to encourage private industry to participate and to justify their fairly risky investment in biodefense product development.

It is my view that Congress did not intend Bioshield to be just another pot of money from which to procure existing drugs, or to only award contracts for new vaccines and therapies to companies and products that have been funded entirely from NIH grants. Unfortunately, it is our view that this is, to a large degree, how the system has played out in the agencies. This has profound ramifications for the future of the Bioshield Program.

However, there is another way: direct that HHS and other relevant agencies to simply implement the law as written.. The federal government would be well served by simply making better use of the authorities the President proposed and Congress has provided and the President proposed in Project BioShield rather than the business-as-usual approach we have seen on ARS countermeasures.

In order for the federal government to more effectively implement the authority and funding it has been granted under Project Bioshield, I would make five main recommendations:

<u>1. Defining markets:</u> In the Bioshield statutory model the government must early on define the market: We will contract for X doses of a drug to respond to Y threat payable upon delivery of an approved product. This is critical because unless the private sector has a clear sense abut what the federal government needs—and what it is willing to buy—the private sector will not invest in the mere hope that the government may one day

procure a certain countermeasure. Absent a defined market, pharmaceutical companies will focus their resources and money in finding new cures for premature baldness, heart disease and erectile dysfunction—drugs they know consumers will buy. In order to harness the ingenuity and resources of the pharmaceutical industry the market needs to be defined and this market needs to provide an adequate return on investment to justify the opportunity costs.

2. Risk and funding: A second key question for the future of Bioshield is who should bear the risk of the drug development process. BioShield was designed to provide early market signals to encourage the private sector to invest in—and bear the risks of—developing new drugs for WMD threats. However, Bioshield has increasingly appeared to be reverting back to a more traditional government-funded research and development program, one in which HHS selects specific grant recipients to fund experimental development efforts.

The risk of this government grant model is two fold. First, only one in ten drug candidates ever receive FDA approval and make it to market. If HHS utilizes Project BioShield to focus on drug development and not procurement, as might appear to be the case thus far, the odds are against picking drugs that will ultimately make it into the Strategic National Stockpile. Second, if HHS picks winners and losers at the early development stage, the industry as a whole will not expend its potentially vast sums of private R&D capital to develop these products for the federal government. Instead, this will become a niche market made up of just a few NIH/HHS companies dependent on federal research grants. As a result, the breadth of technology, knowledge and discovery that will be focused on safeguarding this nation will be only a fraction of what a broader, private sector-based program would provide.

3. Timing and speed: In its May 2005 edition, *Forbes* published an article about the procurement decision to buy a next-generation vaccine for Anthrax. In that article, a former senior-level HHS official from was quoted as saying; "Bioshield was always designed to bring in new products, it was not a piggy bank to buy licensed products." I believe our lawmakers intended Project Bioshield to dramatically speed the development and procurement of new products, by utilizing the law to enter into contracts to procure drugs at an early stage of development. Language from the bill states "potential contractors have to show necessary measures of minimum safety and effectiveness; estimated price for each dose or effective course of treatment regardless of dosage form; and other information that may be necessary to encourage and facilitate research, development, and manufacture of countermeasure or to provide specifications for the countermeasure." Additional language states a countermeasure is available for purchase under Project BioShield if it "is a countermeasure for which the Secretary determines that sufficient and satisfactory clinical experience or research data (including data, if available, from pre-clinical and clinical trials) to support a reasonable conclusion that the countermeasure will qualify for approval or licensing within eight years." Eight years to licensure—that is the statutory standard established by Congress.

However, in all of its Bioshield RFPs to date, HHS has required that products be at the IND stage of development—a relatively advanced stage of development, particularly in the context of WMD medical countermeasures. While there may be valid reasons for HHS wanting to wait to obligate funds for products only after they have essentially been proven after years of early testing and millions of dollars in development costs, this approach is one of the main reasons why there are so few biotech companies now participating in this market space and why there are virtually no large pharmaceutical companies participating at all.

In some respects the department's position seems akin to the Pentagon asking that defense contractors build new ships, tanks and aircraft with only a vague assurance that there will actually be a buyer for them once they are developed and built. Moreover, HHS` apparent concern about spending federal funds on unproven drugs is inapplicable here. Companies that receive an advanced purchase contract under Bioshield only receive payment when the drug is approved and provided to the government. In any case, this approach is certainly no way to build a true biodefense industry in this country.

4. Building market confidence: In the last two-and-a-half years investors have lost confidence in the biodefense industry due to a number of factors. Initially, the long delay in the enactment of the Project Bioshield Act caused a loss of market confidence. Now it is the uncertain, mysterious, and bureaucratic process of securing an actual Bioshield contract that has caused companies, like mine, active in this area to take a beating in their share prices and in their ability to raise additional capital.

We believe this can and must be rectified by a more aggressive, predictable, and transparent Bioshield decision making process. As I mentioned earlier, I fully support efforts to enact a so-called Bioshield II bill, including key provisions to provided needed liability protection and additional financial incentives for companies to develop these countermeasures. However, I also firmly believe that much more can be done today, using existing federal authority and funding, to encourage private sector participation in this arena and to get a host of new countermeasures into the Strategic National Stockpile.

5. Communication: Mr. Chairman, if I had to pick one word to summarize how the Bioshield process must be improved, that word would be "communication." While I realize there are sometimes national security concerns that must be borne in mind when publicly discussing these issues, the fact of the matter is that it has been extraordinarily difficult, if not impossible, to find out anything about this process or about how we, as a small biotech company, might contribute to it. It truly has been a "black box" process, and one that we have had to hire several outside consultants to even begin to understand and participate in. HHS should now publicly indicate the threats for which it intends to buy products, along with reasonable information about the potential size of the order, the requirements for the products, and approximately when the order will occur. And then HHS should affirmatively open a dialogue with the pharmaceutical and biotechnology industries and with individual companies. Without better communication with industry, Project BioShield will very simply fail.

CONCLUSION

For Project Bioshield to be effective and stimulate private companies and investors to participate it simply needs to be implemented the way the law was written. I would encourage HHS, DHS, DoD and the other agencies and sub-agencies involved in this process to reach out even more to their partners in industry. For we are that: partners. We are not competitors with the federal government, nor are we seeking to simply profit from a new source of federal funds.

And I would venture to say that I and virtually all of my industry colleagues engaged in this market space are loyal, patriotic Americans who sincerely want to do our part to enhance our nation's security. We must certainly justify our efforts to do so to our shareholders, but I can assure you and the other members of this Committee that if profit were our only or even our primary motivation, we would have sought other markets or simply abandoned our efforts in this regard some time ago.

The efforts undertaken by this Committee, by Congress as a whole, and by this Administration to bring to fruition innovative new countermeasures are beginning to pay off. While much needs to be done to both clarify and streamline the decision making process. progress does appear to be being made.

Mr. Chairman, distinguished members of the Committee, we are truly on the dawn of a new era with respect to medical countermeasures to weapons of mass destruction. After decades of very little progress from the "duck and cover" days of the early Cold War, we are in the midst of extraordinarily exciting discoveries in vaccines and treatments for a host of man-made and naturally occurring pathogens, from anthrax and smallpox to botulinum and radiation.

The United States has the most innovative, persistent and effective pharmaceutical industry by far of any country in the world, and we have only begun to unleash that amazing potential for the protection of the American people from acts of terrorism. With the continued support and guidance of Congress, and with a Bioshield procurement process that is finally taken out of the shadows, the future could be very bright indeed.

Again, thank you for the opportunity to testify before your distinguished panel today, and I would be happy to answer any questions you may have.

Mr. SHAYS. Thank you, Mr. Hollis. It is an honor to have you here.

Dr. Epstein.

STATEMENT OF GERALD L. EPSTEIN

Dr. EPSTEIN. Thank you, Mr. Vice Chairman and members of the committee.

I do not have a company. I would like to step back a little bit here and discuss some overall aspects of the bioterrorism threat, what those characteristics imply for our ability to counter that threat. I would like to point out that although essential, the programs we have in place are going to be insufficient as time passes on in the long run to deal with threat, particularly emerging threats. And finally, offer some cautions for you to consider.

The bioterrorism threat is real, but it is uncertain in detail. It is getting increasingly more uncertain. Fortunately, we have no historical record to draw from. Moreover, there is no reason to think the future will look anything like the past. We do not know exactly what we are going to be facing.

For one, the technologies involved are what I call pervasively dual use. Essentially every skill, material, piece of equipment or agent one would need to develop a weapon is available and in use somewhere in the economy for a legitimate purpose; not all in one place, but available somewhere. Very little is uniquely malicious.

Second, the technology is expanding both in market penetration and disseminating around the world in ways which will make these capabilities increasingly more accessible to greater numbers of people. Rather than asking the question, will a terrorist really turn to biology and learn something they are not familiar with, we have to recognize that in the world we are headed into there will be more and more people who already know the biology. There the question is, will these people become sympathetic with or turn to terrorism? Learning the technology will not be the problem for them.

Finally, science is continually advancing, realizing more things that we need for beneficial purposes, but opening the possibility of additional ways to attack.

What this means for our ability to counter these threats is that intelligence is going to be able to provide less and less guidance for us to base our planning on. As I mentioned, the dual use nature of the technologies involved means it is going to be very hard to look at something taking place and determine whether or not there is malicious intent behind that.

The expansion into the marketplace and around the world of the relevant capabilities means not only are we looking for a very ambiguous and maybe unknown signal for a weapons program, but we are trying to pull that signal out of a very rapidly growing base of fully legitimate activity. Small signal, large increasing background will make it very hard to use intelligence mechanisms to find out what the problem is.

And as science continues to advance, we may be faced with threats we do not even know today, because we are learning more about how to keep people healthy and unfortunately, how to possibly make them ill.

But the problem is even worse than that. Even if we knew precisely everything about everyone on the planet today that was pursuing malicious applications of biology, the time scales of our defensive preparations versus the time scale of what an attacker would need to go through are quite mismatched. Offense is much more flexible and much more rapid than a defender.

The countermeasures that we need to develop in BioShield and whatever other mechanisms and research approaches we have in place do not need to be focused against the threat today, even if we had a perfect picture of that, but at the threat years down the road when our countermeasures will be deployed. Given the difference in time scales between what it takes to develop a weapon versus what it takes to develop a countermeasure, the threat 5 or 10 years from now may not exist until 4 or 9 years from now. The groups may not be formed, the technologies may not be around.

So in principle, even perfect intelligence about the world today will not be good enough to help guide where we need to go with our defensive efforts.

The BioShield program and the R&D programs at NIH and elsewhere in the Government are essential for countering this threat. But we are going to need a new approach as we look ahead, not a different approach, but additional approaches, as we proceed. For one, we can't just write a list of threat agents and start checking the boxes and going down a list. The vaccine, the countermeasure development programs, are quite expensive. Even $5.5 billion runs out pretty quickly when you spend a half billion a pop.

So some agents are certainly worthwhile focusing on, anthrax and smallpox are so serious and qualitatively enough above other possible threats that it is worth spending a lot of money to deal with those problems. But you can't go very much farther down the list of agents before you recognize that there is not enough money and there are always going to be things you are not going to get to. It is not clear that the ones you have not paid for are less dangerous than the ones you have.

What we need in the future is a broad, flexible and adaptive response capability. This is going to require some new science. We don't really know how to do that now. But it is also going to require some new organizational approaches.

Traditional vaccines, I think, although they are important for the threats we know today, are going to have less and less utility as time goes on. They are too specific. It is too long for them to take effect once they have been administered. And the development process takes too long. We need things like broad spectrum therapeutics and antivirals that can handle several different threat agents that don't have to be designed for a single one.

And then we need a whole set of research tools. We need to improve the productivity and speed of our research and countermeasure development enterprise, assays, screens, computational tools, animal models, ability to predict both, damage mechanism an agent can do, and the ability to predict what a countermeasure may be able to help you with. As we proceed in an era where specific threats will be less and less identifiable, we need that kind of broad capability.

And finally, the caution I would like to hold is, there is certainly and understandably a great reluctance to take Government money and spend it in ways which realizes a private benefit. So there is some interest in saying these are biodefense missions which we need to pursue versus these are commercial interests which we will let the market take place and we don't want to apply Government funds.

As we proceed in the future, it will be harder and harder to tell the difference between a biodefense threat, a biological threat, an emerging infectious disease or another type of natural occurrence. If we design our countermeasures to only handle what we consider to be biodefense but do not address these other areas, we will not be doing the right things.

So rather than avoiding the possibility that we may be actually helping a commercial firm, we actually have to embrace that, I think. I would be glad to answer questions.

[The prepared statement of Dr. Epstein follows:]

Testimony before the
Committee on Government Reform
United States House of Representatives

"BIODEFENSE: BUILDING A MEDICAL COUNTERMEASURE CAPABILITY"

July 14, 2005

A Statement by

GERALD L. EPSTEIN

Senior Fellow for Science And Security
Homeland Security Program

CENTER FOR STRATEGIC AND INTERNATIONAL STUDIES, 1800 K STREET, NW, WASHINGTON, DC 20006
TELEPHONE: (202) 887-0200; FACSIMILE: (202) 775-3199 WWW.CSIS.ORG

Testimony of Dr. Gerald L. Epstein
Senior Fellow for Science and Security
Homeland Security Program
Center for Strategic and International Studies
Washington, DC

Testimony before the Government Reform Committee
U.S. House of Representatives

"Biodefense: Building a Medical Countermeasure Capability"

July 14, 2005

Mr. Chairman and Members of the Committee:

I appreciate the opportunity to appear before you today to discuss the capacity to generate medical countermeasures against biological weapons and bioterrorism. I am currently serving as Senior Fellow in Science and Security in the Homeland Security Program at the Center for Strategic and International Studies here in Washington. I also teach a course on science, technology and homeland security in the Security Studies Program at Georgetown University's Edmund A. Walsh School of Foreign Service. I have been working in the area of science, technology, and security policy for more than twenty years and have been studying biological weapons issues and responses for nearly 15 years.

I spent much of that time working at the Congressional Office of Technology Assessment, where I was project manager for a major series of reports produced for the Congress on the proliferation of weapons of mass destruction, including biological weapons. OTA was eliminated ten years ago this fall, and I cannot resist the opportunity to suggest to the members of this Committee that you and your colleagues would find such a capability to be very helpful in looking at questions such as the ones you are asking today.

At CSIS, my colleagues and I are launching a major international effort, supported by the Carnegie Corporation of New York and the John D. and Catherine T. MacArthur Foundation, to look broadly at biological weapons threats and to identify opportunities to counter them at all stages, from influencing the intent to produce weapons, to denying access to materials and expertise, to detecting illicit programs, to managing the consequences of an attack. We are also looking at perceptions and threat reduction activities across nations and across professional communities. The activities to be addressed at today's hearing are an important part of the United States' – and the world's – response to biological weapons threats.

At CSIS I also organized a workshop to examine the global evolution of dual-use biotechnology, looking specifically at the implications of this evolution for the spread of biological weapons and bioterrorism capabilities (1).

I'd like to spend some time this morning discussing aspects of the bioterrorism threat, what they imply for our ability to counter them, and some high priority actions we need to take as a result. Let me set out the following points:

1) Bioterrorism is a very serious threat, but the details of future biological weapons cannot be known today. Although certain diseases currently pose more serious terrorist threats than others, a wide variety of agents might nevertheless be used, and the exponential growth and dissemination of biotechnology will foster the identification and/or creation of new ones. Since the time to develop and produce bioweapons agents will, in general, be much shorter than the time to develop, license, and produce a response, we will never catch up to the threat if we rely on hard intelligence alone to direct the development of countermeasures.

2) Uncertainties about the future threat put a premium on breadth of capability and speed of response. Looking ahead, the most important medical countermeasures are new "broad spectrum" antibiotic and antiviral drugs and other post-exposure therapies. Traditional vaccines have only a limited role in civilian biodefense, because of the time they need to develop protection; we cannot vaccinate our way out of this problem.

3) Substantially increased NIH biodefense research and the new Bioshield program are necessary components of our national response, but they are insufficient. Further incentives are needed to stimulate production of post-exposure therapeutics and rapid response capabilities, for which we need new research tools and methods. We also need to develop animal models for human disease and increased animal production and testing capacity.

4) Successful incentives that foster biodefense missions could benefit commercial enterprise as well, because many of the necessary supporting capabilities are inherently generic. Policies that attempt to ensure that government incentives or investments apply only to government biodefense missions – as the original version of the first Bioshield legislation attempted to do – are guaranteed to fail at fostering a dynamic, responsive, and flexible biodefense response capability. In the long run, it will be increasingly difficult to distinguish "biodefense" capabilities from broader health-related capabilities, much less target incentives only towards the former.

5) Medical countermeasures are very important, but they are only one component of a comprehensive biodefense strategy. Countering bioterrorism also requires efforts to dissuade, frustrate, detect, and counter bioterrorism programs at every possible stage of their planning and execution, not just after an attack has been conducted.

Characteristics of the Bioterrorist Threat

Importance of Taking the Threat Seriously. As members of this subcommittee no doubt know, history is a poor guide to the bioterrorist threat. There are few areas with so great a gulf between the proven, historical capability to do grievous harm, and the relative paucity of actual attacks.

We know for sure that biological weapons, when prepared for effective dissemination in large enough quantities, can kill over large areas. All the necessary capabilities to place many thousands of lives at risk were demonstrated decades ago. We know that the technology, materials, and expertise required to produce biological weapons are available to those terrorists who are sufficiently motivated and skilled to pursue them; essentially all the equipment, materials, and expertise have legitimate application or can be found without great difficulty. And we know that enemies exist who are eager to kill Americans in vast quantities. What we are not sure of is why we have not yet been attacked in this way. Maybe not enough of today's terrorists took high school biology. Tomorrow's will – and their high school biology classes will be much more potent than today's. We cannot bet our country that whatever restraints have kept terrorists from pursuing this path will persist indefinitely.

Exactly how close terrorist groups are right now to the capability to conduct a major biological attack matters if we want to know how likely it is that such an attack will take place in the near future. However, looking out over the several years that our defensive preparations will take to implement, the details of today's threat are less important than the realization that the rapidly increasing capability, market penetration, and geographic dissemination of relevant biotechnical disciplines will inevitably bring weapons capabilities within the reach of those who may wish to use them for harm (see figure 1).

Difficulty in Predicting or Specifying Future Threats. Given the diversity of potential biological weapon agents and the increasing ability to modify or augment them, either through conventional techniques or genetic engineering, we will never be able to restrict our efforts to a short list of agents considered to be the most serious threats. It is true that certain agents today are considered to pose greater terrorist risks than others because of their combination of health consequences and ease of dissemination. A few diseases, such as smallpox and anthrax, pose such dangers that they are worth special attention (smallpox because of its lethality and contagiousness; anthrax because of its lethality and hardiness). However, a wide variety of agents could be used as weapons, and that list will grow over time as science advances, biotechnology spreads, and new capabilities become feasible.

Intelligence collection efforts will not provide a reliable guide for our biodefense activities. First, the "signatures," or observable signs, of a terrorist bioweapons development activity will be very difficult to detect, particularly amidst a large and rapidly growing background of legitimate biotechnical activities. Bioweapons programs do not require large, expensive, or distinct facilities, and we cannot have much confidence that we will spot them.

More serious is the significant mismatch in time scales between attackers and defenders. Unless we radically transform the way we do business – a scientific and technical challenge as much as a management or resource one -- our programs to design, develop, approve, and produce medical countermeasures will have lead times that are much longer than those of the terrorist weapons programs they are intended to counter. Today's defensive programs cannot be designed against today's threat but rather must anticipate the threat years in the future – posed by groups and programs that may not even exist today. Moreover, we are unlikely to be able to mount major countermeasures development programs covertly. Attackers will probably know what countermeasures we are developing and if possible, will work to evade them.

Implications for Biodefense

Role of Vaccines. Unavoidable uncertainties in the future biological threat place a premium on broad-spectrum, post-exposure therapeutics and rapid reaction capabilities. Traditional vaccines are less relevant, since they are only effective against specific diseases (and often only against specific strains), and because they generally generate immunity too slowly to be of much value if given after the fact. (Smallpox and anthrax vaccines are exceptions, because they have therapeutic value even if given after exposure.) Too many possible other disease threats exist for us to vaccinate our way out of the bioterrorism problem. And we are very unlikely as a society to decide to vaccinate large groups against potential bioterror agents in advance of any attack, since we would not be able to justify imposing the small but nonzero risk of vaccination when we have absolutely no way of knowing what harm – if any -- those vaccines will have avoided.

Novel vaccine approaches – such as so-called "DNA vaccines" – are very important because they offer the tantalizing prospect of mounting an immune response fast enough to have therapeutic value post-exposure. However, such vaccines are too speculative to be able to anticipate successful products, or to fit within the 8-year window needed to qualify for Bioshield I funding. Vaccine research might also lead to the development of antibodies to provide quick but temporary protection against a disease during the time needed for a more conventional vaccine to take effect. Even though these techniques would -- if successful – provide some "post-exposure" response capability, they would still be very specific towards particular diseases.

Need for Additional Antivirals and Antibiotics. Since traditional vaccines are of limited value in responding to an attack, we need antibiotics and antiviral drugs. However, despite their importance for dealing with natural disease outbreaks, let alone bioterror attacks, the development of such anti-infectives has been neglected by the pharmaceutical industry in favor of drugs to treat chronic conditions, such as hypertension, cancer, and heart disease. These conditions provide large and continuing markets, whereas most infectious diseases occur only sporadically, particularly in the developed world markets that can readily afford pharmaceutical products. The required course of anti-infective treatment lasts only a week or two – and if successful it clears up the problem, eliminating the need for further business. Pharmaceutical manufacturers would rather devote their resources to drugs with larger and more lucrative markets -- and they would be punished by their investors if they didn't.

A 2004 paper by UCLA researchers finds that, out of 506 new drug candidates that have been disclosed in the development programs of the largest pharmaceutical and biotechnology firms, only 31 represented anti-infectives: 6 antibiotics; 12 antiviral drugs to combat HIV; 5 other antivirals; 5 drugs to combat parasites; 5 to combat fungi; and 1 other. (2) This dearth of new anti-infectives in the pipeline is especially troubling given the rate at which naturally occurring pathogens are evolving resistance to existing antibiotics and antiviral drugs.

The Infectious Disease Society of America points out that infections that were once easily treatable are becoming "difficult, even impossible, to treat" today. More than 70 percent of the bacteria causing hospital-acquired infections are resistant to at least one of the drugs typically used to combat them. Resistance to multiple drugs is increasing, including resistance to vancomycin, a drug of "last resort." Only two new classes of antibiotic have been developed in the last 30 years. A "class" is a group of drugs that all utilize the same mechanism to kill bacteria or viruses, and that are all rendered ineffective as soon as pathogens evolve the ability to evade that particular mechanism. (3) A 1998 report by the British House of Lords report concluded that "antibiotic resistance threatens mankind with the prospect of a return to the pre-antibiotic era." (4) Clearly there is a critical need for new antibiotics and antiviral drugs, not only for biodefense, but also to combat naturally occurring infectious disease.

Need for Research Tools, Methods, and Infrastructure. In the long run, we need a vibrant, flexible, and responsive biodefense system that can adapt to threats as they materialize. We cannot mount decade-length; billion-dollar scale vaccine or drug development programs to combat every potential threat agent. Therefore, we must develop research tools that can make a much more responsive system possible. Building such a system will be a tremendous challenge, and there are fundamental scientific questions that will need to be resolved. However, there will certainly be need for tools such as assays for rapidly screening drug candidates; improved methods for determining chemical and biological properties of drug candidates that can accelerate and/or replace certain stages of preclinical testing; bioinformatics approaches to identify promising drug targets; and a wealth of other approaches, including many that are undoubtedly yet to be envisioned.

A major component of this research infrastructure will be improved animal facilities and understanding. Given that many diseases of bioterror concern occur too rarely in humans to permit clinical trials, the Food and Drug Administration has specified that efficacy testing of drugs can be conducted in two different species of animals, rather than humans. However, the "animal models" utilized in these tests must be sufficiently well understood so that the drug's effect on the disease in those animals can be reliably related to how that drug would work against human disease. Development of these animal models; as well as the construction of animal facilities in which these animals can be bred and these tests can be conducted, is a critical biodefense need. Right now, shortages of animals, animal facilities, and animal models threaten to constrain research.

Existing Government R&D Programs and Incentives for Industry Are Necessary, but Not Sufficient

The Role of the National Institutes of Health. Substantially increased NIH biodefense research funding, and the Bioshield program that was enacted last year, are both necessary components of our national response -- but even together they are not sufficient to generate these post-exposure therapeutics and other essential components of a response to bioterrorism. Important parts of the problem remain unaddressed, such as the research tools and animal model issues described above.

Scientific investments made by NIH have driven the growth of the biotechnology industry over the last few decades, and the very substantial ($1.7 billion) increase in the level of annual NIH funding for biodefense research will improve our basic understanding of disease pathogenesis as well as lay the groundwork for the development of drug and vaccine countermeasures. These investments are also funding substantial increases in "high-containment" research facilities that allow scientists to work with dangerous organisms safely. NIH has been tremendously productive in its traditional role of pursuing the most exciting and productive biomedical science, leaving industry to pick up and run with what it wants. However, this largely "bottom-up" approach is less well suited for a more mission-oriented, product-focused program to filling specific biodefense needs that involve product design and development, clinical trials, FDA approval, scaleup, and manufacturing. Industry's involvement in this process is critical.

NIH research investments will also be essential for bolstering the scientific underpinnings for improved research tools and methods. NIH has developed guidelines that are intended to ensure that research tools, materials, and other resources developed in the course of NIH-sponsored research become available to other investigators. However, it is not clear that these Guidelines are optimally designed to achieve that end, particularly on the scale that will be needed to support a robust, responsive biodefense capability. The working group that developed those guidelines found that "intellectual property restrictions can stifle the broad dissemination of new discoveries and limit future avenues of research and product development." (5) Although the group also found that "reasonable restrictions on the dissemination of research tools are sometimes necessary to protect legitimate proprietary interests and to preserve incentives for commercial development," (6) the resulting guidelines do not appear to give sufficient emphasis to the role that commercial firms play in improving, standardizing, distributing, and marketing these tools – and to the corresponding ability that these firm must have to control the distribution of the resulting materials and recoup their investment. I hope that other witnesses at this hearing can provide further information on incentives that NIH and others can offer that will best facilitate the development and dissemination of research tools.

The Role of the Pharmaceutical/Biotech Industry. Pharmaceutical and biotech firms, on the other hand, have not in the past had much incentive to develop products for what are essentially government biodefense markets. Debate leading up to the passage of the original Bioshield legislation last year recognized the importance of engaging these firms, the barriers that had prevented them from participating, and the need to develop new incentives to engage them. Indeed, Congress has appropriated $5.6 billion dollars as of Fiscal Year 2004 to fund Bioshield purchases, and procurements using these new authorities are now underway. However, it is not clear that these existing incentives will be sufficient, for example, to motivate firms to increase their development of anti-infectives. Given how important it is to augment our existing antibiotic and antiviral arsenal for public health purposes as well as for biodefense, government incentives to stimulate their development – even ones that are not immediately applicable to biodefense -- would be appropriate.

The original Bioshield legislation also left gaps, such as the failure to provide liability protection for firms that develop medical countermeasures in good faith. The best available scientific and technical understanding notwithstanding, no vendor preparing products to mitigate the consequences of a terrorist attack can ever fully predict the circumstances under which those products would be used, let alone conduct fully realistic tests or evaluations. Nor should products with some potential to mitigate the consequences of an ongoing health emergency or bioterrorist attack necessarily be held to the same standards as products, such as vaccines, that allow a very healthy population to stay that way. It will therefore be important to assure firms that are otherwise willing and able to produce medical countermeasures that the threat of product liability lawsuits will not put their survival at risk. An Institute of Medicine Committee that examined DoD's program to develop medical countermeasures against biological warfare agents concluded that "it is important for the government to address industry concerns about product liability risks as part of efforts to accelerate the development of medical biodefense countermeasures." (7) The SAFETY Act (part of the Homeland Security Act, Public Law 107-296) does provide some liability protection to manufacturers of products to counter terrorist attack, but it does not apply to products used in anticipation of such an attack, as many medical products might be. Nor does it provide compensation for those who may have been harmed by an antiterrorism product. Therefore, if liability protection is to be provided to shield vendors from unwarranted liability claims, some mechanism going beyond the SAFETY Act – and preferably one that provides compensation for legitimate claims -- must be provided.

Inadvisability of Drawing Strict Boundaries between Biodefense and Commercial Missions

At an earlier stage of my career, I directed a study that examined the relationship between military and commercial technologies, looking in particular at the effects and implications of government policies to stimulate one or the other (8).

It was clear at the time -- and it remains true today -- that government policies that have the intent, or the effect, of stimulating commercial technology development can be quite controversial. Legitimate objections would be raised to policies that would put government in the position of "Picking Winners and Losers," with the argument being made that the marketplace was a much more appropriate mechanism than government to make such a determination. Interestingly, I think that "picking winners" was often a bigger problem than "picking losers." The latter merely wasted money, whereby the former took resources from all of us and had the effect of applying them to the benefit of just a few. Even when such actions were well justified on the basis of their public benefit, the fact that there were private beneficiaries raised issues of equity and fairness.

I revisit this debate because I fear that similar concerns could cripple our efforts to generate a vibrant, responsive, and effective biodefense capability. Some of the most important requirements we face – improved research infrastructure; new tools and methods; new antiviral and antibiotic products; new animal models and facilities – are not specific to biodefense; they apply to biodefense and to commercial missions alike. If we are too concerned about "picking winners" – if we avoid taking actions that might benefit commercial firms, even as they support the biodefense mission – we are guaranteed to fail at developing the capabilities we need. The original draft Bioshield legislation ran this risk, since it would have made any product that had a non-biodefense application ineligible for Bioshield support. Congress wisely eliminated that prohibition before enacting that legislation.

Future actions to support our biodefense capability are similarly bound to raise this same question. Given how generically applicable the necessary capabilities are, we must embrace, rather than avoid, these "dual-use" benefits. Clearly, careful attention will have to be paid to the details in any such incentive scheme to ensure that they are not abused by firms that are not contributing to the biodefense mission, or that are taking advantage of loopholes in the procedures to enrich themselves at the public's expense. But if we design a system to prevent firms that support the nation's biodefense mission from realizing benefits in their commercial activities, we are not doing what we need to be doing.

Need for a Comprehensive Approach

Finally, although my comments today have been directed primarily at medical countermeasures to bioterrorist attack, it is important to recognize that we cannot rely solely on after-the-fact responses in dealing with the threat of bioterrorism. As important as they are, medical countermeasures are only one component of a comprehensive biodefense strategy. We must put programs in place to dissuade, frustrate, detect, and counter bioterrorism programs at every possible stage, not just after an attack has already taken place.

One of the chief difficulties in fighting bioterrorism is that none of the measures we can imagine, by itself, can offer high confidence in successfully countering this threat. But by putting a combination of measures in place, or a layered defense – recognizing that each measure or layer has limitations and weaknesses – we can maximize our chances of success.

Endnotes

(1) Gerald L. Epstein, *Global Evolution of Dual-Use Biotechnology: A Report of the Project on Technology Futures and Global Power, Wealth, and Conflict* (Washington, DC: Center for Strategic and International Studies, April 2005)

(2) Brad Spellberg, John H. Powers, Eric P. Brass, Loren G. Miller, and John E. Edwards, Jr., "Trends in Antimicrobial Drug Development: Implications for the Future," *Clinical Infectious Disease* 2004:38: 1279-86

(3) Quotations and statistics in this paragraph from The Infectious Disease Society of America, *Bad Bugs, No Drugs: As Antibiotic Discovery Stagnates ... A Public Health Crisis Brews,* July 2004 (available online at http://www.idsociety.org/pa/IDSA_Paper4_final_web.pdf, accessed February 6, 2005); pp. 9, 10

(4) United Kingdom Parliament, House of Lords, Science and Technology Committee, "Resistance To Antibiotics and Other Antimicrobial Agents," Seventh Report, 17 March 1998, available online at http://www.parliament.the-stationery-office.co.uk/pa/ld199798/ldselect/ldsctech/081vii/st0703.htm (accessed February 6, 2005); section 1.19

(5) *Federal Register,* vol. 64, no. 100 (May 25, 1999), p. 28206

(6) *Ibid.*

(7) Committee on Accelerating the Research, Development, and Acquisition of Medical Countermeasures Against Biological Warfare Agents, *Giving Full Measure to Countermeasures: Addressing Problems in the DoD Program to Develop Medical Countermeasures Against Biological Warfare Agents*, Lois M. Joellenbeck, Jane S. Durch, Leslie Z. Benet, eds., (Washington, DC: National Academies Press, 2004), p. 80 (available online at http://books.nap.edu/books/0309091535/html/80.html#pagetop, accessed February 6, 2005)

(8) Alic, John A.; Branscomb, Lewis M.; Brooks, Harvey; Carter, Ashton B., and Epstein, Gerald L.; *Beyond Spinoff: Military and Commercial Technologies in a Changing World* (Boston, MA: Harvard Business School Press, 1992)

Other Useful References

Bradley T. Smith, Thomas V. Inglesby, Tara O'Toole, "Biodefense R&D: Anticipating Future Threats, Establishing a Strategic Environment," *Biosecurity and Bioterrorism*, Vol. 1, No. 3: September 2003, pp. 193-202

Lynne Gilfillan, Bradley T. Smith, Thomas V. Inglesby, Krishna Kodukula, Ari Schuler, Mark Lister, and Tara O'Toole, "Taking the Measure of Countermeasures: Leaders' Views on the Nation's Capacity to Develop Biodefense Countermeasures," *Biosecurity and Bioterrorism*, Vol. 2, No. 4: September 2003, pp. 320-327

FIGURE 1: Implications of Technology Advance for Bioterrorism

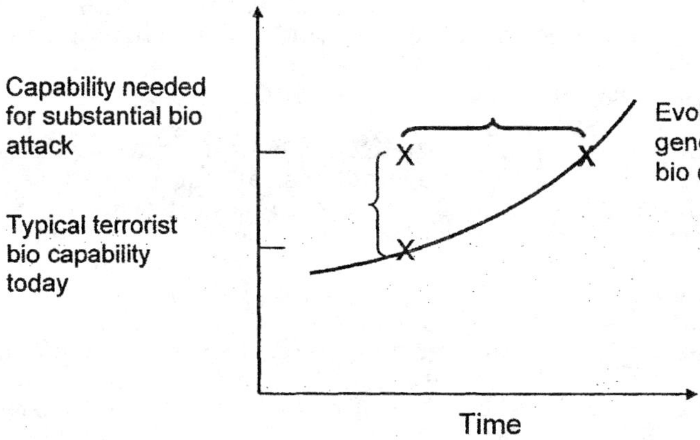

No matter what the actual gap is today between a terrorist group's level of capability in biological weapons and the level needed to do substantial harm, that gap will disappear over time.

Mr. SHAYS. Thank you very much. Thank you, all three of you, for your testimony.

Let me just say that we start with Mr. Issa. We have Danny Davis, Ms. Watson, Mr. Van Hollen and Ms. Norton and then I will ask questions. We will go in that order, unless the chairman comes, and then obviously he will jump in.

Mr. ISSA. It is good to be king, or chairman.

Thank you, Mr. Chairman.

Dr. Epstein, you really made the case for me in your testimony. I was thrilled to hear it. All the problems, all the challenges, all the hurdles and all that we could spend today and it won't fix what is attacking us tomorrow is all true. Conversely, though, once we take the bio out of BioShield, what is left is radiological. I would like you to comment, if you feel I am missing the point here.

But Mr. Hollis, as I see it, if someone goes to an abandoned Russian lighthouse using cesium, that is going to be the same antidote as if they get yellowcake, as if they do a conventional nuclear bomb, as if they do any other kind of dirty bomb. Is that correct?

Mr. HOLLIS. That is correct.

Mr. ISSA. And if another Chernobyl or Three Mile Island were to occur, perhaps because of a terrorist attack, that would be the same antidote, wouldn't it?

Mr. HOLLIS. That is correct. Those isotopes all have major impact on the bone marrow's ability to produce cells that are necessary for health.

Mr. ISSA. And the U.S.S. Ronald Reagan, home ported in San Diego, where I know your company is located, and where I fly back and forth every week, were to have a reactor breach, that would be the same antidote?

Mr. HOLLIS. That is correct. I think what you are getting to is, this is one area we don't have to worry about a different strain or pathogen. We can address this area because of radiation.

Mr. ISSA. So this need has been around and known for non-terrorist activities, but certainly heightened because of terrorist activities since the dawn of the nuclear age?

Mr. HOLLIS. Ever since we split the atom and it was weaponized, yes, sir.

Mr. ISSA. Back to you again, because this really is pivotal to try to look at how much we can do with bio and for how much versus the terrorist and non-terrorist threat that something could happen with radiation. And I might add, somebody mishandling radioactive materials for cancer treatment would be the same, wouldn't it?

Mr. HOLLIS. That is correct.

Mr. ISSA. How far away are you from having a treatment in which somebody will die if they don't get a treatment, how far are you away from having a treatment that could be shown to be effective?

Mr. HOLLIS. We got clearance through the FDA and we are scheduled to perform our pivotal efficacy trial the second half of this year. We are in the current process right now of setting that trial up. Concomitantly, we are also setting up our human safety trial, so we could actually have an NDA through the FDA by 2006.

Mr. ISSA. And the standard that the FDA normally uses, as I understand it from my time at Energy and Commerce, is two-fold.

One, you have to have minimal adverse side effects and two, you have to work, you have to be better than nothing at all. Is that also applied to your potential treatment through the FDA?

Mr. HOLLIS. With weapons of mass destruction in June of last year, the FDA passed the animal efficacy rule, where it is unethical to expose human beings to, for instance in this case, lethal doses of radiation. You can get approved using the animal efficacy rule in relevant animal species, in this case, non-human primates. You have to establish safety in human beings. That is the regulatory process that we are going through.

We have been developing this product exclusively for the past 3 years and the Armed Forces Research Radiobiology Institute started researching this product back in 1997. So this product has been in the process of being developed for the past several years. We believe if we stay on course, because of the major investment our corporation put into it, that we can have a licensable product by the end of next year.

Mr. ISSA. So the end of 2006?

Mr. HOLLIS. Yes, sir.

Mr. ISSA. And yesterday we had former speaker Newt Gingrich and others in to talk about entrepreneurship and people, the Government having a process in which it did not take the risk but rather transferred the risk to the private sector, to entrepreneurs who would take that risk in return for a return.

As I understand, there have been no Government dollars to do this development. This has been on the back of your public company stockholders, is that right?

Mr. HOLLIS. That is absolutely correct. Maybe this is an opportunity I can say that, what I have been hearing today with the first panel is not what I am experiencing in reality. I am starting to wonder, sir, if they have read the same BioShield legislation that Members of this Congress passed. Because it is not being implemented the way it has been written. Companies like ours were supposed to get advanced purchase contracts and paid on delivery.

Mr. ISSA. I ask unanimous consent for 2 more minutes.

Mr. HOLLIS. So it is not being implemented, nor are entrepreneurs being rewarded for the risks they are taking. We are a role model for BioShield. We are executing it according to the way it was written, and that is, private investment capital pursuing these markets that were supposed to be guaranteed markets. And after 3 years of development, we don't even know what our market is yet.

Mr. SHAYS. I am going to allow the gentleman to go 2 more minutes and allow 7 minutes for everybody.

Mr. ISSA. Thank you, Mr. Chairman.

You are a public company, is that right?

Mr. HOLLIS. That is correct.

Mr. ISSA. So the money, I appreciate it is private sector, but the money that you have used, how much has it been approximately, just roughly?

Mr. HOLLIS. Approximately in this technology, in the product, about $150 million.

Mr. ISSA. And that came from public stock?

Mr. HOLLIS. All investors, yes.

Mr. ISSA. So would it be fair to say that your fiduciary obligation to the market, and for that matter, Bill Arak and others who sue people when they foolishly abuse the public stock market, depends on a good faith belief that if you make this product, the Government has committed to purchase it, if it works, if it is the most effective, there was a commitment for that in BioShield.

Mr. HOLLIS. That is absolutely correct, and we are developing the drug according to the way the legislation was drafted and passed. It is just not being implemented that way. So if there are shareholders that end up getting concerned about it, I think these things will start to come into question.

Mr. ISSA. My time has nearly expired. I am sure that there will be followup along this line.

Dr. Epstein, I appreciate your being used, in a sense, to prove the point. But I would also reiterate that with the complexity, with the number of needs that are going to happen on the bio side, I think it is important that we take this one item and say, are we, and this is what government reform is all about, are we meeting our commitment so that hundreds of potential products, people are going to spend billions of dollars developing them, when we are the most likely customer, based on a good faith that if we need them, and if we say we want them, that we will then make a good faith purchase if they are developed and if you are the winner of that process, recognizing not everyone will win.

And with that, I yield back, Mr. Chairman.

Mr. SHAYS. Thank you very much. Thank you, Mr. Davis, for your patience. You have the floor for 7 minutes.

Mr. DAVIS OF ILLINOIS. Thank you very much, Mr. Chairman.

Mr. Hollis, I guess I could probably glean from your testimony that there have been some rather frustrating and costly delays, that it is costing perhaps not only your company but others frustration, but also uncertainty, relative to the development of product that could be moved to the point of procurement that we greatly need. Would that be an accurate assessment of the description of what I have heard?

Mr. HOLLIS. Yes, sir, that is absolutely correct.

Mr. DAVIS OF ILLINOIS. If that is the case, and given that as the case, is there a way that these developments can be structured so that of course, any time one ventures into something that is new and perhaps different, there is a certain amount of risk. And there is a certain amount of risk taken. I guess there is also a certain amount of risk sharing.

Is there a way to make sure or to try and make sure that the risk is such that the American public, that is the Government, and those who are willing to, on the other hand, invest their resources, can have the assurances that both are being protected and that is a win-win situation or a model that is going to produce a win-win situation for both parties?

Mr. HOLLIS. Yes, sir, there absolutely is. No. 1, industry would ask that the Project BioShield legislation be implemented as it was drafted and passed by Congress. I truly believe that the individuals who are implementing it have made up the rules as we go along. Because if you read the legislation, it is about stimulating capital formation and biotech and pharmaceutical companies to produce this Nation's next generation medical countermeasures to mitigate the medical consequences of weapons of mass destruction.

And to unleash the ingenuity of the entire pharmaceutical industry, it means it has to put the market incentives in place, and it needs to execute the legislation as it was written.

What is happening here is most of the medical countermeasures that are being produced are NIH or AID funded. Those are the products that seem to be getting the attention.

So if that is the case, why would the pharmaceutical industry engage? The pharmaceutical industry just needs to know what the rules are and have them implemented. When BioShield was initially passed, many people in this industry were excited to produce the next generation medical countermeasures. The fact that it has been implemented with a lack of leadership and a lack of implementation and sense of urgency and a huge sense of bureaucracy has basically killed the capital markets and the ability to raise money to develop these drugs.

So if the capital markets and the companies that want to participate in this area are not incentivized, all the medical countermeasures are going to be dependent upon the NIH and taxpayer dollars. So to answer your question, BioShield II would be great. But I think most importantly, BioShield II needs to be implemented the way it was crafted.

Mr. DAVIS OF ILLINOIS. It could be that there might be opportunity for a different level of consultation with the industry or with the pharmaceutical industry as the rules are being shaped, realizing that again, both sides have to be comfortable as well as protected, and of course, the American public is always afraid that somebody is going to get a windfall out of something. So you don't want that to happen, either.

Would a different level of consultation perhaps be helpful in the process?

Mr. HOLLIS. Possibly more open dialog, clear transparency and guidelines, so that the people implementing the bill are directly interfacing with industry representatives, so the process is transparent and everyone knows what is expected of one another. If we are expected to be partners with the Government to develop these medical countermeasures, then we need to be treated as partners. There needs to be that dialog.

Also, sir, I don't believe there is windfall. I believe that if you are developing a medical countermeasure and spending your investor dollars and taking those risks, and if your technology is good enough to get FDA approval, and it can safeguard and protect the American people and provide these medical countermeasures, those companies should win.

Mr. DAVIS OF ILLINOIS. Thank you very much, Mr. Chairman. I have no further questions.

Mr. SHAYS. I thank the gentleman.

Ambassador, thank you for your patience.

Ms. WATSON. Thank you, Mr. Chairman.

I think this goes right to the heart of the comment I made about our responsibility here to have the oversight to address the issues that you are raising, Mr. Hollis. Are we providing the opportunity or are we going along with the provisions in the BioShield Act to be sure it is implemented?

I think Dr. Epstein raises our vision on this whole thing. Are we preparing for the moment? Are we laying an infrastructure for the future? Every day something new occurs around this globe. I am sure the threats are turning inward now. I have no doubt in my mind that we will not witness some kind of biochemical attack.

I had an interesting experience coming in from Cuba. After I got through Customs, the Customs agent ran behind me and said, were you recently in the hospital? Yes, I had some nuclear exams, and they picked up the radiation as I came through. Blew my mind. I saw little red and amber and green buttons flickering, but I did not know what it meant.

So I think it makes the case that we have to expand our vision and we have to do oversight to see that we are getting what we ask for. So I would like first, Dr. Epstein, to comment on what Mr. Hollis has presented to us in terms of what their company has been doing, thinking that Government would keep its word and allow the marketplace to compete and do the research. Dr. Epstein.

Dr. EPSTEIN. I am not familiar with the details of Mr. Hollis' case.

Ms. WATSON. You don't have to be, but you hear the issue he is raising.

Dr. EPSTEIN. Certainly the intent of the legislation was to stimulate our private enterprise, recognizing that the biotech and the pharmaceutical industry had not worked very closely with the national security community. And it by and large did not like Government money very much.

So this mechanism was trying to stimulate a market which would provide incentives closer to what they already operate on and I think it is a very important question to investigate how well the intent and the wording of that legislation is actually being implemented.

I am also struck by Dr. Fauci's remarks earlier. Mr. Hollis has a product, so the development work has been done. If we are starting with a need, I wish I had something to cure such and such, and then you are starting out doing the science, we are a very long way away.

As Dr. Fauci pointed out, even doing the research may not get you to the range where you can use the BioShield mechanism, because we have to have an expectation within 8 years we will have a useful product. And there may be some development work between the research that tells you, here is a possibility, and the certainty that lets you know that within 8 years, we think we can invest our funds, or a company can invest our funds and get there.

I have heard some attention paid to this gap between that. And I think that bears looking. There may be a need for something besides NIH funding, besides BioShield to try and bridge things.

The last thing I would like to add if I may is, on the question of how general versus how specific countermeasures are, and I just want to get back to the question Mr. Issa asked on radiation countermeasures, it is true that one possible source of radiation is a source outside, other than x-rays or gamma rays will irradiate people. In that case, an x-ray is an x-ray, so a countermeasure that protects against that will be helpful against anything.

Another type of radiation exposure is when there is contamination that you breathe or you eat. That makes a tremendous difference in what it is, because if it is radioactive iodine, it will go to the thyroid, if it is radioactive strontium, it will go to your bones. There the countermeasure makes a great deal of difference.

So the fact that we have potassium iodide to protect against some isotopes in nuclear power plants will do essentially nothing for a radioactive dispersal device. And one has to worry about both of those. So you need the general case, but also recognizing that there are specifics.

Mr. HOLLIS. If I may answer part of that question.

Ms. WATSON. Please, Mr. Hollis.

Mr. HOLLIS. Dr. Epstein brings up a very interesting point that is unrelated to radiological countermeasures. However, it is a point worth noting, because our company was founded on the premise that there are hormones that are signaling agents in the body that can stimulate innate and adaptive immunity. We actually started out in infectious diseases, we have conducted multiple phase two clinical trials in HIV/AIDS, tuberculosis and malaria. We have established the fact that the product is active in all three areas. It is the one drug for many bugs.

We were looking at a broad spectrum approach to infectious diseases over a decade ago. I have spent 30 years in this industry, and I realized that we were running into problems with resistance to antibiotics and resistance to infectious diseases. Our whole core technology platform was based on stimulating innate and adaptive immunity.

We have not even brought this technology to BioShield. It is actually a true bioshield. It is not going to be a cure for everything, but it is certainly a very active drug that can be used to probably defend against multiple pathogens.

But why isn't that product being targeted for BioShield? Because they have not identified a market for a broad spectrum drug that would work against many pathogens or developed the models that we can put our drug in to see if they work. There needs to be better vision in regards to where we are taking BioShield in the future. So I absolutely agree with Dr. Epstein and his broader vision, because we share it.

Ms. WATSON. Thank you so much. I would like to address a comment and question to you, Mr. Kramer. You testified that the Department of Health and Human Services has contracted to purchase 5 million doses of BioThrax, the licensed anthrax vaccine manufactured by your company. You also stated that without a firm commitment from the Department to purchase additional quantities, it may be difficult for you to keep BioThrax production facilities up and running.

Obviously the Government faces a difficult task in deciding which biodefense products to purchase for the National Stockpile, and in what quantities. As we have already heard today, a bioterrorist attack could come in the form of a number of different agents, including ones that we cannot foresee today.

Yet we must be ready now with access to sufficient quantities of best measures currently available. This is the tension that the Department must manage on a day to day basis. I would ask you about your ability to keep manufacturing the BioThrax without further commitment from the Department to purchase additional quantities. I think that is where Mr. Hollis was going with his testimony as well.

Mr. KRAMER. Certainly. Let me try to touch on all those, starting with your question in terms of how do we establish the sense of accountability for how BioShield is being implemented. I think you really need to separate questions of science, as you heard some of the earlier panel members talk about, versus policy. And it is not my position necessarily to second guess the scientific decisions that are being made by Dr. Fauci's group or other people in a place of authority or responsibility for that.

But I would question the policy that is being implemented. I think this is where my suggestion that the scientific advisory committee or some group can certainly help you all with that. On the policy side, it is pretty easy to get your arms around what is being done strategically in terms of how we are addressing these threats.

We have signed a contract with HHS for 5 million doses of our product. We are partially through the delivery of that order, probably a couple million doses into that. We have not supplied all of those 5 million doses. But I think it is important to understand that it has taken HHS almost 3½ years to pull the trigger on putting the first dose of licensed product into the stockpile, and that did not occur until 2 months ago.

So my concern is from a policy perspective, given the challenges of operating biologic facilities in this increasingly compliant world. Your question about how long are we willing to continue to do this without a firm commitment from the Government, that is a very touchy issue. We have been at this for almost 7 years now since acquiring the facility in 1998. We have always put the U.S. Government's requirement or potential requirement for BioThrax front and center in terms of all the customers. We have looked at selling the product commercially, both to foreign governments as well as to other domestic customers. But we have always placed the U.S. Government need for the vaccine first.

So obviously, we want to make sure that we are responsive to that need. We also need to look at the commercial markets for the product and beyond that we will have to make a very simple business decision whether it pays for our shareholders to continue to operate a facility at significant cost on an ongoing basis when there is not a commensurate commitment by the Government to order vaccine.

The other issue that I will say is——

Mr. SHAYS. I need you to kind of shorten up your answer.

Mr. KRAMER. OK, just one last point. There is very clearly an acknowledged threat regarding anthrax. HHS and other folks have determined that they need 75 million doses of vaccine in the stockpile today to protect Americans. Why are they not buying as much of our product as possible while the experimental products and new technologies, which are years away, have a chance to even prove that they are going to be successful? That is my issue.

Ms. WATSON. I know my time is up, Mr. Chairman.

Mr. SHAYS. If you have another question, go for it.

Ms. WATSON. I want to go through the Chair to Dr. Epstein. I was very intrigued by your testimony, because you had the broader vision. And I was hoping that we as a committee, subcommittee, would request you to do a paper specifically on what we need to do to meet the intent of the BioShield Act that you feel is needed. Apparently the policies are not being implemented according to our intent.

And I would like to see, Mr. Chair, if we could ask Dr. Epstein to submit to us a paper—now, I tried to read through his testimony, but there is so much there. Maybe you can specifically give us some guidance and direction.

Mr. SHAYS. That is a fair request. I don't know how much time it would take you to do it, but the pay is good. [Laughter.]

Dr. EPSTEIN. I will certainly try and be responsive. It is a tremendously broad question. But if there are a few insights I can offer you, I will be happy to submit that.

Mr. SHAYS. Yes, maybe you can narrow it down a bit.

Dr. EPSTEIN. Mr. Chairman, on this point, I put this in my written statement, I refrained from saying it orally, but I cannot resist this opportunity. The experience I have worked on in biological weapons and biological proliferation I did as a member of an agency which worked for you, which worked for the U.S. Congress. I was at the Office of Technology Assessment, working on biological weapons issues.

That office was closed 10 years ago this fall, and I think for precisely the reason you brought that question up, you don't just need an individual behind a desk giving you individual views. I think you need an institution, you need a group of people that work for you and answer precisely that kind of question without any allegations of working for anybody else. I think that is something you could very much use.

Mr. SHAYS. Thank you very much.

I am going to yield my time to Mr. Issa and let him ask some more questions.

Mr. ISSA. Thank you, Mr. Chairman. I will be brief. I would like to follow on what my colleague from California, Ms. Watson, had started on. This is the, no surprise to you, this is the committee on Government Reform. We are an interesting committee, because we are mostly about oversight, unless it comes to where Government is not doing what we have already asked them to do. Then suddenly we are a relatively, if not a very powerful, committee.

I think that we have hit on something here, I think Ms. Watson even made it clearer, it appears as though we have some specific problems in implementation of the law and for what reason is the question that I am going to leave you with. You will have time to answer, don't worry about those bells or the man behind the curtain.

It appears to me, and I would like your comments and you are free to disagree with me, it appears as though if you work with NIH, if you are an organization in-house or out of house, but you are already being funded by us, that you have the inside track on follow-on solutions. If you are completely an outsider, meaning truly entrepreneurial and not entrepreneurial with Government assistance already, that you are on the outside and at a disadvantage.

Now, that seems to be Mr. Hollis' statement, that this is part of this, now we are going out fishing for something when a product has already gone through part of the FDA process, and it probably should be more about, is there any other product that is this far along, because we need something sooner, not later, as we were told by the earlier panel.

Is this your observation? I guess to each of you, but Dr. Epstein? And you don't have to be bad-mouthing the Government, but is there an advantage inherent that is part of the problem?

Dr. EPSTEIN. I think part of what makes working for the Government difficult is that those who have done it before always know that system better. Part of what BioShield wanted to do was to open that up more broadly.

But I think again, taking a bigger view, many of the things we are going to need to do nobody does. So it won't be a matter of whether there is an existing contract or a new startup. It is going to be all new. So it is an interesting question, do the big pharmaceutical firms who have not been terribly interested to date, are there additional incentives one can offer them to bring them in, or is that a group which is not really nimble and flexible enough to do what we need, and we have to go to a different strata?

So I think we have to recognize that track records are important. But we also have to recognize that there may be things for which there is no track record.

Mr. ISSA. Mr. Hollis.

Mr. HOLLIS. I think there are degrees to what I testified to and to what your comments are about possibly some conflicts. Because if you do receive a grant you are in and there is a lot of communication and dialog. If you don't have a grant, you are depending on the legislation to be implemented, because that is why a company like ours participates in it.

So the oversight is extremely important, because I think the committee would do themselves well to re-read the legislation and ask yourselves, if you were industry, how do you interpret this. Because obviously, there is a misinterpretation in regard to how it is written, how it is being implemented. And if the pharmaceutical industry is going to participate in this, and that is what the legislation is drafted and passed and designed to do, then it really needs to examine how it is being implemented.

Mr. ISSA. Mr. Kramer.

Mr. KRAMER. I think certainly there is a clearer risk that happens. One can only look at how HHS announced the first contract under BioShield to VaxGen when they very systematically laid out how the award of an $877 million contract to this company was the prototype of how BioShield should work, meaning you had intellectual property which was developed at USAMERID early on, it was transferred to NIAID for mid-stage development and then it was procured under BioShield. They trumpeted that loud and clear, that was the poster child for how BioShield moneys were to be spent.

And while that may work in some instances, it should not be the only way that BioShield works, which I think is what my colleague Mr. Hollis and I are both saying, is that's not the only way it could work. Because industry is looking at the Government very closely to see how they are acting in relation to BioShield. And when they smell that there is something untoward going on, they will be very cautious about investing their shareholders' capital in areas of risk where there is not commensurate return.

Mr. ISSA. Mr. Chairman, I think that gives us a pretty full picture. Our work is cut out for us. I would yield back.

Mr. SHAYS. Thank you, all three of you, for your testimony. I just would say, if you have a 30 second ending that you just want to put on the record, we will be glad to hear it. Otherwise, we will adjourn. Is there any closing comment that any of you would like to make?

Mr. HOLLIS. Maybe I can start. I would just please ask the committee to really use your authority in looking at the oversight of the implementation of this. We would really like to see BioShield work. It is important for this country's safety and security. I think it is the best way to produce medical countermeasures, and that is unleashing the industry and innovative entrepreneurs and new approaches to diseases, with the full realization that unless we get FDA approval and we deliver, the Government is not obligated to pay us anything.

Mr. SHAYS. I think we got your message. And I think you can be pretty sure there will be good followup.

Mr. HOLLIS. Thank you.

Mr. SHAYS. Dr. Epstein.

Dr. EPSTEIN. I'm not taking my shot, Mr. Chairman.

Mr. SHAYS. OK, thank you. Mr. Kramer.

Mr. KRAMER. Just one last comment, and that is, I think it is critically important for there to be a higher degree of oversight and accountability by the Government agencies in terms of following through with BioShield. They need some help in terms of early and mid-stage review of these critically important products. Otherwise you are not going to get that well-rounded, mature, biodefense industry that is going to be a partner to the Government in the long term.

Mr. SHAYS. Thank you, that is a nice way to end. We will conclude this hearing. Thank you, gentlemen.

[Whereupon, at 1:50 p.m., the committee was adjourned.]

[The prepared statements of Hon. Christopher Shays, Hon. Darrell E. Issa, Hon. Jon C. Porter, Hon. Carolyn B. Maloney, Hon. Elijah E. Cummings, Hon. C.A. Dutch Ruppersberger, and additional information submitted for the hearing record follow:]

ONE HUNDRED NINTH CONGRESS

Congress of the United States

House of Representatives

COMMITTEE ON GOVERNMENT REFORM

2157 RAYBURN HOUSE OFFICE BUILDING
WASHINGTON, DC 20515–6143

MAJORITY (202) 225–5074
FACSIMILE (202) 225–3974
MINORITY (202) 225–5051
TTY (202) 225–6852

http://reform.house.gov

SUBCOMMITTEE ON NATIONAL SECURITY, EMERGING THREATS,
AND INTERNATIONAL RELATIONS

Christopher Shays, Connecticut
Chairman
Room B-372 Rayburn Building
Washington, D.C. 20515
Tel: 202 225-2548
Fax: 202 225-2382

Statement of Rep. Christopher Shays
July 14, 2005

Project BioShield represents a critical tool in the war against terrorism. A flexible, streamlined capacity to identify, develop, procure and stockpile medial countermeasures means our response can be as dynamic and agile as the threat we face.

So it is important to measure the pace and trajectory of the BioShield effort one year later. Is the program achieving the goal Congress intended - to draw private sector partners into the risky development of vaccines and therapeutics we hope no one will ever need to use? Are we more secure against the threat of biological terrorism than we were a year ago? How do we stay prepared against a rapidly evolving threat? And how does BioShield assess the risks of endorsing the use of untested medicines against unknown threats?

During House debate on the BioShield bill, I expressed concern over provisions allowing the use of unapproved vaccines and treatments by military personnel. Testimony before the National Security Subcommittee by Gulf War veterans confirmed the Department of Defense (DOD) had consistently failed to meet basic requirements to inform recipients about investigational drugs or keep adequate medical records.

The mandatory DOD anthrax vaccine program only built on that sorry record, relying on a dated vaccine formulation tested and approved only for protection against cutaneous exposure, not against weaponized, aerosolized anthrax. A federal court has enjoined use of the vaccine in a mandatory program due to flaws in the Food and Drug Administration approval process.

But, rather than rely on BioShield to develop a modern anthrax vaccine, the Pentagon chose to rely on another provision of the law permitting the Department of Health of Human Services (HHS) to grant "emergency use authorization" for continued use of the now "unapproved" anthrax vaccine, albeit in a voluntary program. At the time, I expressed my concerns about the request, about DOD characterization of the alleged emergency and about the rigor of the process used by HHS to grant this precedent-setting authority. It appears the matter was given little more than a cursory, uncritical review. I still have questions about the adequacy and wisdom of that decision, questions I hope can be addressed today.

Recent reports indicate less than half of US military personnel have agreed to take the anthrax vaccine, a clear indication our troops are carefully weighing the benefits and risk of the vaccine. The process for approving the use of unapproved, untested medicines should be no less thoughtful.

DARRELL E. ISSA
49TH DISTRICT, CALIFORNIA

WASHINGTON OFFICE:
211 CANNON HOUSE OFFICE BUILDING
WASHINGTON, DC 20515
(202) 225-3906
FAX: (202) 225-3303

DISTRICT OFFICE:
1800 THIBODO ROAD, SUITE 310
VISTA, CA 92081
(760) 599-5000
FAX: (760) 599-1178

SOUTHWEST RIVERSIDE COUNTY
(951) 693-2447

www.issa.house.gov

Congress of the United States
House of Representatives
Washington, DC 20515–0549

COMMITTEE ON GOVERNMENT REFORM
SUBCOMMITTEES:
ENERGY AND RESOURCES—CHAIRMAN
FEDERAL WORKFORCE & AGENCY ORGANIZATION

COMMITTEE ON INTERNATIONAL RELATIONS
SUBCOMMITTEES:
INT'L TERRORISM & NONPROLIFERATION—VICE-CHAIRMAN
EUROPE & EMERGING THREATS
MIDDLE EAST & CENTRAL ASIA

COMMITTEE ON THE JUDICIARY
SUBCOMMITTEES:
COURTS, THE INTERNET & INTELLECTUAL PROPERTY
IMMIGRATION, BORDER SECURITY & CLAIMS

HOUSE POLICY COMMITTEE

July 14, 2005

Introduction of Richard Hollis

Thank you, Mr. Chairman.

Mr. Chairmain, I would like to introduce to the Committee one of our witnesses this morning, Mr. Richard Hollis, Chairman and CEO of Hollis-Eden Pharmaceuticals, which is located just north of San Diego and very near my congressional district. It's an exciting company that seems to have tapped into a potentially huge new area and direction of medicine—that of managing the human body's immune system and how it responds to certain diseases and challenges, like radiation exposure. This could have huge implications for how we treat a number of diseases, including those potentially caused by weapons of mass destruction.

Mr. Hollis first came to see me almost two years ago to tell me about an exciting radiation sickness drug that they were developing and to explore whether and when the federal government might be inclined to purchase such a drug under Project Bioshield. This is after he had apparently already been at this process at the various agencies in charge of this program for at least a year.
And here we are today, almost three years later and four years since the 9/11 attacks and the federal government has still not moved to stockpile a radiation sickness drug, although I understand that there are some signs that that may soon be in the works.

Mr. Hollis continues to believe that the only way this Bioshield program will work is with the involvement and participation of the private sector, particularly among smaller, biotech companies like his that are willing to venture out into this fairly new and somewhat risky field of WMD medical countermeasures. I tend to agree with that assessment, Mr. Chairman, and I hope that the testimony and discussion this morning bears this out. Because without this participation, and without a clearer path for companies like this to take in trying to offer such products to the federal government, Project Bioshield simply will not work.

In any case, I, along with several of our colleagues, introduced the Radioprotectant Procurement Act of 2005, which essentially mandates that the federal government move on this issue and procure one or more radiation sickness (radioprotectant) drugs within a specified time frame. This could be this drug or some other drug—the bill is obviously neutral on that point. But what the bill does make clear, as does a letter to Secretary

Leavitt, Mr. Chairman, that you and I and 14 of our colleagues who recently signed the letter, is that having an appropriate emergency and medical response and plan in place to respond to a nuclear or radiological attack deserves a much higher priority than it has apparently gotten thus far among the agencies charged with this responsibility.

We read virtually ever day about how the proliferation of nuclear materials and technology threatens to make 9/11 look like a "toothache," to borrow a phrase from a recent author on the subject, Professor Graham Alison at Harvard. Yet the priority in terms of procuring medical countermeasures seems to continue to be anthrax and smallpox, as well as other pathogens.
And while these are no doubt real and important threats, I think any rational analysis of the issue indicates that such attacks would pale in comparison to a nuclear bomb being detonated in New York or Washington or San Diego. Again, I look forward to the testimony this morning and of hearing a clear and specific plan from our government panel as to how we are going to prepare for the unthinkable should it happen on our soil.

Thank you, Mr. Chairman, and thank you for appearing today before us, Mr. Hollis.

STATEMENT FOR THE RECORD
CONGRESSMAN JON C. PORTER (R-NV-3)
"One Year Later: Evaluating the Effectiveness of Project Bioshield"
July 14, 2006

Thank you, Mr. Chairman, for holding this hearing today. I would also like to thank the witnesses for being here to provide the Committee with an update regarding Project Bioshield.

Last week, we were reminded of the evil intentions of terrorists throughout the world. The tragic bombings in London just go to show how far certain individuals will go to harm others—a tragic commentary of the world we live in today.

Now that we have experienced terrorist attacks on airlines, buses, and trains, it is imperative that we work to ensure that terrorists are deterred from using chemical or biological attacks within our homeland. In order to protect our citizens from the spread of biological agents, such as anthrax, and serious diseases, such as Ebola and the plague, Congress authorized the Department of Health and Human Services (HHS) to implement Project BioShield to help secure medical countermeasures against a biological attack.

As you described, Mr. Chairman, Project BioShield gave the government the ability to develop and purchase vaccines and other drugs to protect Americans from a bioterrorism attack. Within the last year, HHS has awarded contracts to private companies in order to create vaccines for biological agents such as anthrax—a positive step for this young program.

Mr. Chairman, I firmly believe that proactive, as opposed to reactive, measures with respect to bioterrorism are the best way to protect our citizens. I look forward to hearing the testimony from our witnesses, and I thank you for holding this hearing today.

***

Representative Carolyn B. Maloney (NY-14)
Project BioShield
July 14, 2005

I would like to thank Chairman Davis
and Ranking Member Waxman
for holding today's hearing
about the effectiveness of Project BioShield.

Given the serious threat of bioterrorism,
the development of effective countermeasures
to biological agents is vital
to our national security.

The goal of Project BioShield must be
to encourage the development of these projects.

Most of us vividly remember
the anthrax attacks of October 2001
including the fear they caused
about the dangerous consequences of exposure.

"The Project BioShield Act of 2004"
was signed into law to enhance the nation's

response capabilities in the event
of a biological attack.

I know that we all agree
that we need to take the appropriate steps
before an attack occurs, if it occurs,
so that we are prepared to treat those
who may be exposed
and prevent widespread illness and death.

As we move forward and consider changes
to Project BioShield,
it is imperative that we review
what has happened
since its enactment one year ago.

Our constituents deserve our attention
and vigilance on this issue
so that they will have confidence
in the safety of themselves, their families,
and their communities.

I thank the witnesses for appearing
before the committee,
and I look forward to hearing their testimonies.

Thank you.

Opening Statement

Representative Elijah E. Cummings, D-Maryland

Hearing Entitled: "One Year Later: Evaluating the Effectiveness of Project BioShield."

Committee on Government Reform
U.S. House of Representatives
109th Congress

July 14, 2005

Mr. Chairman,

Thank you for calling this critically important hearing to assess the implementation of Project BioShield.

The tragic events of September 11th illustrated in no uncertain terms the grim reality of terrorism. In the post 9/11 world, our nation must be fully prepared to not only provide substantial improvements to aviation security, but also to effectively and efficiently address the emerging threat of bioterrorism.

Such preparedness begins by ensuring the federal government has ready access to effective countermeasures to biological, chemical, radiological, or nuclear agents. Regrettably, while considerable progress in recent years has been achieved in the development of treatments to diseases that have a commercial applicability, the development of effective countermeasures to a bioterrorist incident has in large part been stifled due to little private market demand for such products as anthrax vaccines and potassium iodide.

To counteract this troubling situation, Congress passed with my support, the Project BioShield Act. This legislation seeks to encourage and hasten the research, development, and acquisition of effective countermeasures for the Strategic National Stockpile (SNS) that can respond to a bioterrorism attack.

It is vitally important to the health and welfare of our citizens and our nation that Congress rigorously evaluates whether the enhanced authority and funding being utilized under Project BioShield is effective. In practice, the Secretary of Homeland Security designated that smallpox, anthrax, botulinum toxin, and radiation and nuclear devices represent significant threats to the United States.

While Project BioShield is in the process of acquiring a variety of countermeasures against such threats, only three countermeasures have been procured. They include: a pediatric version of a nuclear countermeasure, a VaxGen anthrax vaccine for $878 million, and the licensed anthrax vaccine for $122.7 million.

While Project BioShield represents in many ways a step in the direction toward increasing our nation's biodefense preparedness, I am nonetheless concerned with a central aspect of Project BioShield's implementation.

Unfortunately, despite the financial incentives set forth under Project BioShield, large pharmaceutical companies with extensive research and development budgets, and a thorough understanding of how to navigate the regulatory process have remained largely uninvolved. During a Congressional hearing in 2003 Michael Friedman, PHARMA's Chief Medical Officer for biomedical preparedness, stated "it is necessary to recognize scientific, legal and economic impediments to the research and development of biodefense products."

While we must seriously consider proposals that would help overcome these barriers through additional incentives, we need to be especially attentive to avoid any unintended consequences that would result in higher drug prices and needlessly high payouts to large drug companies with little to show for it.

One need not be an expert to comprehend the magnitude of the loss of life and the disastrous impact a large scale bioterrorist incident would cause to our economy and society. Mr. Chairman, our nation must be ready to safeguard our citizens by providing them with the proper treatment in the event of a bioterrorist attack. Any less would be an abdication of our responsibility to protect our citizens from threats both seen and unseen.

I yield back the balance of my time and look forward to the testimony of today's witnesses.

Congressman C.A. Dutch Ruppersberger
Committee on Government Reform Oversight
Hearing

"One Year Later: Evaluating the Effectiveness of Project Bio Shield"

July 14, 2005

Statement:

Thank you Mr. Chairman for holding this oversight hearing entitled "One Year Later: Evaluating the Effectiveness of Project Bio Shield."

One year later, the country is better prepared than ever to meet the threat of terrorist attack with biological, chemical, radiological or nuclear agents. The national stockpile of medical countermeasures is more extensive and can be accessed more rapidly than ever, and additional diagnostic tests, drugs and vaccines are currently under development.

However, my concern is the possibility of the intentional use of biological or other dangerous pathogens that represent a threat to our society.

Unfortunately, the medical treatments available for some types of terrorist attacks have improved little in decades; however there has been tremendous and rapid progress in the treatment of many serious naturally-occurring diseases.

The major concern that I have with all of these potential attacks on our society is "Are we preparing for the correct attack?" I have said this statement in a previous hearing because my concern is "What else is out there that we are not focusing on?"

While it may be true that the President believes in bringing researchers, medical experts, and the biomedical industry together in a new and focused way, it is my belief that our Nation can achieve the same kind of treatment breakthroughs for bio-terrorism and other threats.

Although, I understand the purpose of the "Project Bio Shield Act of 2003" my concern is making sure that the citizens of the United States always are protected and kept informed as we continue the fight on terrorism.

By discussing how to best examine the efficiency and effectiveness of countermeasures among government defense and health agencies, I hope to be given a clear understanding of where we are in terms of combating some of these major threats.

We need to look at the wider spectrum here and be clear at what we are looking for when it comes to these vaccines and other drugs to protect Americans in the event of a bioterrorist attack.

My concern and commitment will always be the welfare of this nation and continuing to put this effort at the forefront of our nation will only help us to understand our constant threat of attacks.

I look forward to hearing the testimony presented today and I look forward to asking questions of the witnesses.

Thank You.

TESTIMONY OF LANCE GORDON, Ph.D.

CHIEF EXECUTIVE OFFICER AND PRESIDENT
VAXGEN, INC.

SUBMITTED FOR THE RECORD
TO THE
UNITED STATES HOUSE OF REPRESENTATIVES
COMMITTEE ON GOVERNMENT REFORM
HEARING OF JULY 14, 2005

"One Year Later: Evaluating the Effectiveness of Project BioShield"

REGARDING THE IMPLEMENTATION OF PROJECT BIOSHIELD AND THE STATE OF BIODEFENSE IN THE UNITED STATES

Mr. Chairman, Ranking Member Waxman, members of the Committee, I am pleased to submit testimony to the Committee for the record regarding the implementation of the Project BioShield Act of 2004 and VaxGen's role in our nation's preparedness to respond to an anthrax attack as the recipient of the largest contract to date under Project BioShield.

Before turning to the substance of my testimony allow me to thank the Chairman, the Ranking Member and the rest of this Committee for your longstanding efforts to better protect this nation against the threat of bioterrorism. Your leadership is vital to safeguarding the American people.

My name is Lance Gordon; I'm President and CEO of VaxGen. I bring to VaxGen more than 20 years of experience in the vaccine industry, developing both vaccine products and companies. Prior to joining VaxGen, I served as CEO and a member of the Board of Directors of two vaccine companies; OraVax and North American Vaccines. While at OraVax, I was responsible for the organization and initiation of a 20-year program that supplied a stockpile of smallpox vaccine to the Centers for Disease Control for civilian biodefense. I am the inventor of ProHibit® for infant meningitis, the first bacterial conjugate vaccine to receive FDA approval, and led efforts that created a new vaccine licensed by the FDA for whooping cough. I was recently appointed to the National Vaccine Advisory Committee (NVAC). NVAC advises and makes recommendations to the Department of Health and Human Services (HHS) on issues related to preventing infectious diseases through immunization.

VaxGen, Inc. is a California-based biopharmaceutical company focused on the development, manufacture and commercialization of biologic products for the prevention and treatment of human infectious disease. Founded in 1995, one of VaxGen's business strategies emphasizes the development and commercialization of vaccines for the prevention of potential bioterrorism threats, specifically anthrax and smallpox.

VaxGen: A Contractor's View of the Implementation of Project BioShield

We believe VaxGen can offer a unique perspective on the implementation of Project BioShield since our company was awarded the first and to date, the largest contract under the law. Overall, we believe that insofar as the anthrax vaccine contract is concerned, Project BioShield has been successful. The procurement process has led to close cooperation between our company, HHS, FDA, and the NIH. It will yield an anthrax vaccine that is superior to the current one in terms of cost, safety, purity, efficacy, efficiency and administration. We believe many aspects of the process followed and the outcomes achieved should serve as a model for future procurements under Project BioShield. Additionally the challenges encountered and addressed in the process should inform future procurements under Project BioShield.

Let us provide the Committee with a brief history of how we came to win this contract. On November 4, 2004, VaxGen won a competitive bidding process and was chosen by HHS to receive an $877.5 million contract to supply 75 million doses of a new generation, recombinant technology anthrax vaccine known as recombinant Protective Antigen or rPA, for the nation's civilian Strategic National Stockpile. The multi-year competitive process we participated in to win the anthrax vaccine contract was thorough and exhaustive.

As Stewart Simonson, Assistant Secretary, HHS Office of Public Health Emergency Preparedness, testified before the Senate Appropriations Committee on April 28, 2005, "HHS defined a three-stage development and acquisition strategy with open competition for awards at each stage. The early and advanced development programs were supported by the National Institutes of Health's (NIH) National Institute of Allergy and Infectious Diseases with contract awards in September 2002 and 2003, respectively. These were milestone-driven contracts with well-defined deliverables including the manufacture of clinical-grade vaccine and the conduct of Phase 1 and Phase 2 clinical trials. Large-scale manufacturing capacity would be required to support the civilian requirement for this medical countermeasure, which was defined through an interagency process to be the initial protection of up to 25 million persons. Senior officials throughout the United States government evaluated acquisition options to achieve this requirement and, in the fall of 2003, the decision was made to pursue the acquisition of rPA anthrax vaccine."

The Project BioShield contract award we won last November followed on the heels of two competitive anthrax vaccine development contracts awarded to VaxGen by the NIH in successive years: an approximately $21 million development contract awarded in 2002 and an approximately $80 million development contract awarded in 2003. The decision to award each of the contracts to VaxGen included consideration of specific information on our candidate vaccine and our performance under preceding contracts. This history gave the government direct insight into the extent to which they could rely on our candidate vaccine and upon our ability to perform under the contracts.

The competition in which VaxGen participated was an open government procurement process, conforming to all applicable rules and regulations, in which any qualified bidder could participate and several did. We believe the government chose VaxGen among several competing bids because of the advanced development status of our candidate vaccine, our demonstrated manufacturing capacity and the proposal we submitted, which was judged to be superior on technical, cost and scientific grounds.

We are extremely proud to be developing the vaccine designed to protect millions of Americans in the event of an anthrax attack. This is a hugely important role and we're passionate about our commitment to assuring the public's safety and national security. We are pleased that Project BioShield allocated the funds that enabled us to win this contract to help our nation respond to the threat of bioterrorism.

Reasons for Procuring a New Anthrax Vaccine

Why did the U.S. government decide to procure a new anthrax vaccine? The answer is because the Institute of Medicine (IOM) recommended that was the prudent thing to do. In its 2002 report, "The Anthrax Vaccine: Is It Safe? Does It Work?," the IOM stated, "...the committee is convinced that relying on AVA (the earlier generation anthrax vaccine) and the current specifications for its use is far from satisfactory. There is a need for research toward the development of a different and better anthrax vaccine, as well as a need for improvements in monitoring the safety of the current vaccine.... The committee concludes...that ***a new vaccine***, developed according to more modern principles of vaccinology, ***is urgently needed***."

This vaccine also fulfills one of Project BioShield's primary goals, to encourage deployment of the 'best in class" countermeasures at competitive prices." We believe VaxGen's new recombinant vaccine will be "best in class", including attributes such as consistent purity, safety, efficacy, ease of administration, state of the art manufacturing processes and price, demonstrating that HHS's procurement process under Project BioShield has clearly been a success with regard to the anthrax vaccine. Let me briefly share some thoughts with regard to these attributes:

Safety and Consistency

VaxGen's rPA102 vaccine is composed of a single well-defined protein, Protective Antigen, known to be the basis of protection against inhalation anthrax. VaxGen's product specifications call for 95 percent purity. Modern recombinant technology has allowed VaxGen to consistently produce the vaccine at nearly 100 percent purity – significantly higher than what can be obtained using older technologies.

To date, VaxGen's anthrax vaccine is proving itself to have less reactogenicity than AVA. There have been no serious adverse safety events related to VaxGen's anthrax vaccine in either of our clinical trials. These trials included approximately 600 people and the first of the two trials compared our vaccine with AVA. The essential results of both of these trials were reviewed by the Office of Research and Development

Coordination in the Office of Public Health and Emergency Preparedness at HHS, the National Institute for Allergy and Infectious Diseases and the FDA prior to the contract award.

Efficacy

VaxGen's first study in humans, designated VAX005, was designed to determine the initial safety and immune response to its rPA102 vaccine. At FDA's suggestion, an AVA control group was included to make sure that the level of immunity stimulated by our vaccine was "in the ballpark" of that induced by AVA. As part of the study protocol, only two doses of AVA, separated by one month, were administered to subjects in the AVA control group.

The results of VAX005 have been publicly presented by our independent investigators at the International Conference on Emerging Infectious Diseases in Atlanta and the American Society of Microbiology's Biodefense Conference in Baltimore. All doses were safe, and, after the first two doses of AVA or rPA102, the highest two rPA102 doses, 50 and 75 mcg, showed toxin neutralizing antibody responses similar to the AVA group. Toxin neutralizing antibody is the only efficacy parameter in humans accepted by the FDA, as it directly measures the ability of the immune response to the vaccine to neutralize or inactivate the anthrax toxin.

Another important observation suggested that, after two doses of either rPA102 or AVA, immune responses were similar and after the third dose of rPA102, toxin neutralizing antibody levels were higher than the levels achieved after two doses of AVA.

Administration

VaxGen's vaccine is being developed to protect before and after exposure to inhalation anthrax and is designed to require only a few doses for protection. VaxGen's rPA102 has also been designed to provide long-term protection following three doses administered over six months or less. Furthermore, the rPA102 vaccine is the first anthrax vaccine being developed specifically for prevention of inhalation anthrax, the most likely form of the disease to be used as a weapon of bioterrorism.

Cost

We believe that one of the positive features of Project BioShield's first procurement effort is that it will save the government money. Having one company produce all 75 million doses of anthrax vaccine will be a significant cost savings for the taxpayers. VaxGen can deliver its vaccine for $11.70 per dose due to economies of scale. A full course of immunization (3 doses) of VaxGen's vaccine costs $35.10, while a full course of AVA (6 doses) costs $150, or four times as much. Obviously, the savings can be spent on other, much-needed biodefense countermeasures.

Finally, I would also like to take the opportunity to comment on the issue of single source. As you know, representatives from both the private and public sector ask the question whether having a single supplier of the new anthrax vaccine poses supply problems like those that plagued the flu vaccine.

The answer is unequivocally no. Making the flu vaccine and the anthrax vaccine are two very different undertakings. With the flu vaccine, the vaccine virus is grown in live chicken embryos and a company has only one chance to get the vaccine right. It has to be redeveloped every year to make accommodate new production strains of the vaccine virus. VaxGen's manufacturing process is based on tightly controlled large scale cell culture which would be consistent year to year, producing a vaccine that will have a shelf life of several years.

In the case of an anthrax vaccine, a single supplier eases the distribution in the event of another anthrax attack. Just imagine the difficulties of trying to direct panicked civilians to choose among different anthrax vaccines in the middle of an attack when they live in the same city or different cities. Developing clinical evidence supporting interchangeability of different anthrax vaccines would also be prohibitively expensive and time consuming.

Having multiple companies simultaneously developing similar products for the same market also creates a strain on limited resources that could slow vaccine availability and jeopardize availability of countermeasures. There is limited capacity for conducting critical and pivotal animal efficacy studies in compliance with Good Laboratory Practices regulations, as well as limited availability of highly qualified clinical investigators and insurance industry capacity to provide adequate product liability coverage.

When VaxGen bid on the BioShield anthrax vaccine contract, it is important to note that our proposal offered HHS the option that we would share our technology with another manufacturer to establish a second source of supply, an offer that still stands today. However, they asked that we delete that portion of our proposal, presumably because of the advantages of having a single supplier.

In conclusion, we'd like to emphasize to this Committee that Project BioShield is a valuable tool in helping our country defend itself against the threats posed by bioterrorists. VaxGen is proud to have received the very first contract under Project BioShield and is honored to play a critical role in our nation's defense. Producing a vaccine that can save lives, reduce suffering and help protect our country from attack is a source of pride for our company. While our excellent partnership with the HHS, FDA and NIH is a first for our industry, we have made huge progress in a very short time and we are committed to produce and deliver a vaccine in almost half the time of the normal regulatory pathway, regardless of what challenges may lay ahead.

Statement for the Record by Dr. Andrea Myerhoff

Before the United States House of Representatives

Committee on Government Reform

Oversight Hearing: Implementation Project BioShield

July 14, 2005

Medical Countermeasures for WMD Defense: Strengthening the BioShield Process

Mr. Chairman and Members of the Committee, thank you for the chance to submit to you the findings of a Scientific Advisory Panel convened by industry to look at activities of the first year of the BioShield program. I am Dr Andrea Meyerhoff, an infectious disease physician who has previously served the federal government as the FDA's Director of Counterterrorism and then as the Pentagon's Director of Medical WMD Defense. I am an Associate Professor of Clinical Medicine at Georgetown University. Today I represent an international panel drawn from science, public health, and industry to evaluate the BioShield program with focus on an individual product, the anthrax vaccine. Our analysis has driven us to a more general conclusion that can enhance protection of the public health and encourage industry involvement in this important program. With the benefit of the perspective of one year of operation of BioShield, we recommend that the program be strengthened with the establishment of a science-driven, systematic, open advisory process to weigh the complex risks and benefits of medical countermeasures proposed to protect the US population from WMD threats.

Background

The panel I speak for today was convened by BioPort Corporation to independently evaluate and issue its opinions regarding the BioShield program and anthrax vaccine. We closely examined the government's decision to procure an investigational, recombinant anthrax vaccine to fulfill 93% of the anthrax vaccine requirement for the Strategic National Stockpile (SNS). Because of the structure of BioShield, which has the laudable goal of speeding the development of needed countermeasures, this early stage vaccine was procured while still unproven, and while there is available a well-studied, FDA-licensed vaccine. What became clear in the course of our analysis was that the issues raised by this procurement have far broader application than it might appear. How indeed do we evaluate the prospect of a new countermeasure to protect the public health from a WMD threat when there already exists an approved, well-studied countermeasure for the same purpose? And similarly, what is the acceptable risk-benefit balance of a new countermeasure when there is no other for that purpose? We believe these complex questions are best addressed by an impartial science-based process that draws on many relevant areas of subject matter expertise. Such a process would be conducted openly, much the same as we see with a number of Advisory Committees convened to aid the federal government in important public health decisions such as approval of drugs and vaccines by the FDA.

The need for such a process for biodefense products is particularly acute because federal public health planning, rather than traditional market forces, drives the development of medical countermeasures. And while regulation by FDA addresses some issues specific to medical biodefense countermeasures, its regulatory mandate does not extend to others. Because decision-making for WMD preparedness is a complex process with such important consequences, we recommend the creation of a panel with scientific, public health, industry, legal, and public policy expertise to advise government planners on procurements of medical countermeasures for WMD. The aim is provide an open forum for evaluating such countermeasures with regard to safety, efficacy, availability, and precedent. Specific examples from the BioShield process regarding anthrax vaccine will illustrate each of these points.

Medical Countermeasures for WMD:

The Issues at Stake- Safety, Efficacy, Availability, Precedent

Safety: The safety of vaccines is evaluated in both pre- and post-market testing. The established anthrax vaccine has been well-studied; it is perhaps one of the most scrutinized in vaccine history. Over 5 million doses of this vaccine have been administered to more than 1.3 million people. It has been the subject of more than 20 post-marketing studies. Information from the manufacturer of the investigational new anthrax vaccine suggests it has been studied to date in 500-600 people. Rigorous pre-marketing safety trials, which generally enroll thousands of subjects, have not always told the entire story. A recent example illustrates this point. The recombinant Lyme disease vaccine was licensed by FDA in 1998. Pre-marketing human trials enrolled approximately 10,000 subjects. Nineteen months after licensing and the distribution of 1.4 million doses, questions arose about the possibility that the vaccine could exacerbate or cause arthritis. Though a causal relationship could not be established, persistent concerns about this safety issue coupled with poor sales resulted in withdrawal from the US market in 2002.

This example illustrates how the large post-marketing database is the ultimate measure of a vaccine's safety. Accrual of such a safety database is a slow and uncertain process for biodefense products, which raises the question of how best to determine whether there is a need to replace existing, traditionally manufactured, FDA-licensed WMD countermeasures with investigational ones. This raises complex questions that extend beyond the customary dialogue between the manufacturer and the regulatory authorities:

- What will be the size of the pre-market human safety database required for a new vaccine for use in the highly specialized circumstances of a biological release?
- How will the needs of the SNS be met if a significant safety issue is discovered late in the development of a single-source vaccine?
- When considering the use of a new countermeasure, when an established countermeasure is already available, how much safety data is enough?

Efficacy: Unlike the more commonly used vaccines, the efficacy of biodefense vaccine candidates cannot be tested in humans. Traditionally, clinical efficacy testing relies on the case-control field trial, which compares natural infection rates between vaccinated and unvaccinated individuals and is usually the pivotal test for licensure. Indeed for the established, FDA-licensed anthrax vaccine, efficacy was demonstrated in case-control studies at a time when certain factory workers were at risk for occupational exposure to anthrax. However, today biodefense vaccines cannot be tested these ways because natural human exposures to such biological agents are rare, and it is unethical to intentionally expose humans to biological agents such as anthrax. Therefore, efficacy testing of most biodefense vaccine candidates will require alternative regulatory mechanisms that include the use of animal models ("Animal Efficacy Rule"). The accuracy of such models for predicting human efficacy depends importantly on the similarity of the disease and the immune response in animals as compared to humans. Gaps in the knowledge of this comparison make prediction of human efficacy difficult. In the case of most public health vaccines there are ongoing opportunities to assess their performance in controlling infectious diseases. In contrast, for a new anthrax vaccine there is not the opportunity for such ongoing evaluation, and there may only be the very real test. This raises certain questions:

- When an FDA-licensed medical countermeasure that has been studied in humans is available, what information is necessary to determine the efficacy of an experimental countermeasure, which cannot be studied in humans, to be assured that the public will be protected from a potentially fatal disease?
- Should a different standard of efficacy other than the existing regulatory standard of demonstration of non-inferiority be applied to a new product when an existing product meets the current need?
- How will the needs of the SNS be met if a significant efficacy issue is discovered late in the development of a single-source vaccine?

Availability: Like safety and efficacy, vaccine manufacturing facilities are regulated to a high standard. The importance of consistency of manufacturing and its possible effect on product availability is perhaps best illustrated by the serious and unexpected shortage of influenza vaccine in the US during the 2004-05 flu season. This resulted from manufacturing problems with the company contracted to provide approximately 50% of the nation's needed stockpile of flu shots. This shortage illustrates the critical importance of sourcing biodefense medical countermeasures from reliable and multiple suppliers. Under the current structure, approximately 93% of the SNS need for anthrax vaccine is to be supplied by the manufacturer of the experimental anthrax vaccine. The need for medical countermeasures in the event of a biological threat raises the following questions, best addressed by an advisory panel that includes the highly specialized knowledge of manufacturing and distribution found only in industry:

- What kind of availability should be demonstrated by a manufacturer of a new countermeasure when an FDA-licensed product is already available?
- How will the needs of the SNS be met if there arises an availability problem with a single source manufacturer?
- How does the government ensure availability of supply from more than one supplier to avoid risks associated with manufacturing or other supply problems or delays?
- Can industry maintain a warm-base for manufacturing WMD countermeasures without a contract for procurements from the US Government?"

Precedent: Anthrax is the first of many biothreats for which policy makers will need to evaluate the relative risk and benefit of established versus new products before committing public funds to protect the public health. The issues I've outlined here are some of the many that are best addressed by the kind of process we advocate. Such a process can guide subsequent federal public health decisions when the procurement of a new medical countermeasure is contemplated in the setting of an established one. Indeed, aspects of it are applicable to the evaluation of procurements for medical countermeasures that are 'first in their class,' an equally complex question though perhaps with a different risk-benefit equation.

Conclusion

In the biodefense arena, historical market forces are superseded by government decision makers. And quite appropriately there is an interest in new technologies. Issues of safety, efficacy, availability and precedent raised in the analysis of anthrax vaccine procurement are applicable to the wide range of WMD medical countermeasures considered for the BioShield program. The complexity of such important decisions requires a science-based, systematic, impartial process to evaluate the relative risks and benefits of current and new medical countermeasures. We recommend the appointment of a panel of government, academic and industry scientists, lawyers and public policy makers to drive an impartial process for informing government decisions regarding expenditures for medical WMD countermeasures.

I appreciate this opportunity to submit this testimony to you today. Thank you.

APEX
TP
9780160751509
76901953-2